TRANSITIONING FROM LPN/VN TO RN

▼ ▼ ▼ ▼ ▼ ▼ ▼

Moving Ahead in Your Career

Gena Duncan MSEd, MSN, RN

Associate Professor of Nursing
Ivy Tech State College
Fort Wayne, Indiana

René DePew MSN, APRN

Assistant Professor of Nursing
University of Saint Francis
Fort Wayne, Indiana

THOMSON
━━━━━━★━━━━━━
DELMAR LEARNING   Australia   Canada   Mexico   Singapore   Spain   United Kingdom   United States

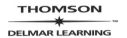

Transitioning from LPN/VN to RN
Moving Ahead in Your Career
By Gena Duncan and René DePew

Vice President Health Care Business Unit:
William Brottmiller

Editorial Director:
Cathy L. Esperti

Acquisitions Editor:
Melissa Martin

Editorial Assistant:
Patricia Osborn

Marketing Director:
Jennifer McAvey

Senior Production Editor:
James Zayicek

Developmental Editor:
Maria D'Angelico

Library of Congress Cataloging-in-Publication Data
Duncan, Gena.
   Transitioning from LPN/VN to RN : moving ahead in your career / Gena Duncan, René DePew.
      p. ; cm.
   Includes bibliographical references.
   ISBN 1-4018-1087-X
   1. Nursing. 2. Nursing—Vocational guidance. 3. Career development. I. DePew, René. II. Title
   [DNLM: 1. Career Mobility. 2. Nurses. WY 16 D911t 2005]
   RT82.D86 2005
   610.73′06′9—dc22   2004049373

$\mathscr{C}$ontents

▼ ▼ ▼ ▼ ▼ ▼ ▼

PART I: ROLE TRANSITION

$\mathscr{P}$reface

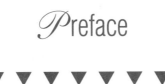

The authors applaud the LPN's/VN's decision to seek new educational goals. This book was written to assist the LPN in making a smooth transition to the RN role. The text addresses the theoretical nursing concepts in meeting the needs of the LPN to associate degree nursing student in a straightforward, easy-to-understand manner. Because of the multiple variations in LPN education, a variety of conceptual and clinical areas are addressed—including math review, intravenous (IV) therapy, care plan development, and assessment skills—that the LPN will need in smoothly transitioning to the RN role. The text assists students with organizing study skills and life responsibilities. Credibility is given to both LPN and RN roles. The changes that the LPN is expected to encounter in the transition from the LPN to the RN role are thoroughly explored. Nursing theory is discussed, and the role of the RN in research is explored. Important concepts such as integration and application of the nursing process and Gordon's functional health patterns are discussed.

Drawing from their backgrounds in LPN and ASN education, the authors address the student's socialization needs in transitioning from the LPN role to the RN role. Faculty teaching LPN-RN courses and former LPN-RN students were surveyed to determine needs of LPNs as they make the transition into RN programs.

$\mathscr{O}$RGANIZATION OF THE TEXT

The professional requirements needed for the RN role are divided into four parts: "Role Transition," "The Nurse as Caregiver," "The Nurse as Manager," and "Professional Considerations." "Role Transition" prepares the LPN student for the return to school by reviewing basic study skills and strategies; identifying individual learning styles; and suggesting time-management skills in balancing the responsibilities of home, work, and school. This part further explores the change process in transitioning and socializing into the new RN role. The student is skillfully guided through reading and critical thinking activities to take a candid look at the LPN role and the RN role in an objective, nonconfrontational manner.

The topics in "The Nurse as Caregiver" prepare the LPN for expanded roles and responsibilities in clinical judgment; problem solving; decision making; client teaching; and communication skills with colleagues, clients, and in crisis situations.

In "The Nurse as Manager," the roles of the nurse as a leader and manager are explored, with emphasis on delegation, accountability, time management, conflict management, decision making, and resource management. The roles of leader and manager are defined and explored.

Finally, in "Professional Considerations," the student reviews the nurse practice act in relation to the scope of practice and explores the legal and ethical issues in nursing by reviewing personal value development and ethical decision making. Major nursing concepts are discussed and nursing theories are briefly presented, with a direct exploration and practical presentation of how nursing theory directly relates to nursing practice.

In these chapters, LPNs are encouraged to grow as they explore the personal changes they can anticipate in the educational process. New concepts are presented in the text so that LPNs can objectively explore their current thinking about the role of the LPN versus the RN and then slowly begin to internalize the RN role. Critical thinking activities appropriately placed throughout the chapters allow the LPN to rethink present views and reflect on new concepts.

Key information regarding math review, clinical assessment, NCLEX review using the new question format, and IV therapy skills is placed in the appendixes to address a variety of needs.

FEATURES

Each chapter includes learning objectives, a list of key terms that are boldfaced and defined in the text, and highlight boxes containing key chapter concepts. A scenario representing the chapter content is followed by "Think About It," questions to center the students' thinking on the content. The chapter themes are further developed by a brief discussion of the content followed by critical thinking activities that assist the students in rethinking the content and developing their personal beliefs about content. At the end of the chapter, students are drawn back to the scenario with "Chapter Reflections," questions that guide them to internalize the RN role both personally and socially. The critical thinking activities present surveys, self-evaluation tools, and charts to accommodate different learning styles. These activities can be used individually by the student or in group discussions in class or on-line.

$\mathscr{A}$BOUT THE AUTHORS

Gena Duncan has two master's degrees, one in secondary education and the other in community health nursing. She taught LPNs for 15 years at Ivy Tech State College and then took a teaching position at Lutheran College that had an ASN and BSN completion nursing program. After Lutheran College was acquired by the University of Saint Francis, she was director of its ASN program. During this time, she guided the curriculum development of an LPN-ASN transition program. She now is an associate professor in nursing at Ivy Tech State College and teaches in the ASN program, where an LPN-ASN program will be starting in fall 2005. Throughout her career, she has taught LPN, ASN, BSN, and master's level students.

René DePew began her nursing career as an LPN in 1987 and moved on to obtain her BSN in 1998 and then her master's, as a family nurse practitioner, in 2000. She is currently assistant professor of nursing at the University of Saint Francis (Fort Wayne, Indiana) in the ASN and BSN programs. She teaches a medical surgical course to ASN and LPN-RN students, and an introductory nursing course to BSN students. She also serves as faculty advisor to the student nurses association.

$\mathscr{C}$ONTRIBUTOR

Chapter 10, Nursing Theory as a Basis to Practice Nursing, was written by Julie Barnett BSN, RN, Assistant Professor of Nursing, University of Saint Francis, Fort Wayne, Indiana.

$\mathcal{A}$CKNOWLEDGMENTS

The authors wish to thank:

Julie Barnett for her assistance in writing the chapter scenarios.

Maria Gomez and Heather Krull for their candid answers to transition issues they personally made in advancing from LPNs to RNs.

Dick Stump for his art concept suggestions.

Mary Spath for her invaluable input in the needs of LPN-RN students. She teaches a transition course for LPN-RN students at the University of Saint Francis in Fort Wayne, Indiana.

Kim Penland for her input regarding the needs of an LPN transitioning into an RN program. She began her nursing career as an LPN and now has her MSN.

Maria D'Angelico for her attention to text content and detail. She has been a tremendous support in the completion of this text.

$\mathcal{A}$VENUE FOR FEEDBACK

We value your feedback and questions, suggestions, or comments about the text. You may contact the authors or publisher at:

Gena Duncan: e-mail: gduncan@ivytech.edu; phone: 260-480-4284 or 260-480-4271

René DePew: e-mail: rdepew@sf.edu; phone: 260-434-7633 or 260-434-3239

Thomson Delmar Learning
5 Maxwell Drive
Clifton Park, NY 12065

$\mathscr{P}$ART I
Role Transition

▼ ▼ ▼ ▼ ▼ ▼ ▼

$\mathscr{C}$hapter 1
Returning to School

▼ ▼ ▼ ▼ ▼ ▼ ▼

$\mathscr{L}$EARNING OBJECTIVES

By the end of this chapter, you should be able to:

1. Discuss phases students experience throughout the education process.
2. Explain four learning styles.
3. Discover your individual learning style.
4. Identify specific time-management skills.
5. Identify study skills to assist in the education process.
6. Discuss ways to balance home, work, and school responsibilities.

$\mathscr{K}$EY TERMS

Abstract random (AR)
Abstract sequential (AS)
Concrete random (CR)
Concrete sequential (CS)
Conflict phase
Honeymoon phase
Learning style
Resolution phase
Returning to School Syndrome (RTSS)
Time management

$\mathscr{S}$CENARIO

Megan has been an LPN for five years. She is planning to go back to school to obtain her associate degree in nursing (ASN). Megan works full-time and has two school-age sons, Todd, age 9, and Shane, age 13. Her husband, Jim, travels quite frequently for his job. Megan feels that studying will not be a problem for her because she can study at her children's games, on her work breaks, and in between her other various activities.

$\mathscr{T}$HINK ABOUT IT

1. How does your own schedule compare to Megan's schedule?
2. How many hours do you anticipate that you will need for school obligations?
3. Does Megan's schedule seem realistic to accomplish her educational goal?

$\mathscr{I}$NTRODUCTION

According to a study by Green (1996), licensed practical nurses/licensed vocational nurses (LPNs/LVNs) who chose to pursue a higher degree have frequently received excellent work reviews for nursing competence and critical thinking. These students were successful not only in completing their degrees but in passing state boards and obtaining jobs.

The fact that you are enrolling in school to earn an associate degree demonstrates your commitment, desire to learn, and ability to set personal and professional goals. You have given much thought and personal analysis to this decision. Perhaps you experienced some self-doubt and anxiety. However, a stimulating, enriching experience awaits you in pursuing an associate degree. This will be an adventure of personal and intellectual growth. Many emotions may already have surfaced, and you will experience many more in the next few months as you pursue your educational goal. In an article entitled "Be a Real Survivor," Melissa Ezarik (2001) states, "Take the challenge, and you'll reap the rewards."

In this chapter we will discuss coping skills that will assist you as you pursue your associate degree. You will be introduced to the Gregorc learning styles and given time-management techniques to improve your study habits. Helpful suggestions will also be given for balancing the demands of school, home, and work. Many of these suggestions may not be new to you, but they will serve as reminders to guide you through future successful semesters.

*D*EVELOPING A POSITIVE ATTITUDE

The three phases of the Returning to School Syndrome (Shane, 1983) are the honeymoon phase, the conflict phase, and the resolution phase.

By reviewing experiences other students have had as they went through the educational process we may gain insight into ways to cope successfully and avoid some undesirable diversions. In 1983 Donea Shane described the emotional ups and downs students experienced when they returned to school for an associate degree and termed the experience the **Returning to School Syndrome (RTSS)** (see Figure 1–1). During the **honeymoon phase,** the student is fascinated with all the new aspects of academic life. There is an increased awareness of purpose and confidence to achieve. This phase lasts until the student encounters a class with in-depth nursing theory or clinical experience. When this occurs, the student experiences anxiety, may feel intimidated, and dreads the clinical evaluation.

The second phase is called the **conflict phase.** During this time, new and different nursing concepts are presented and the student experiences conflict with various personal roles, faculty members, and previous knowledge base versus newly acquired knowledge. The student experiences uncertainty and self-doubt and may become angry, feel overwhelmed, and be fatigued. The institution, faculty, home life, or any tangible object may be blamed for the lack of perceived success. This phase is divided into two parts: *disintegration* and *reintegration.* During disintegration the student turns anxious feelings inward and becomes depressed and withdrawn. In reintegration, the student shows feelings of frustration by acting hostile toward others, especially the faculty. The student expresses feelings of frustration with the nursing program and the education process in general.

The student realizes that her previous knowledge and experience base does not have to be destroyed but is one on which a solid, expanded educational foundation can be built.

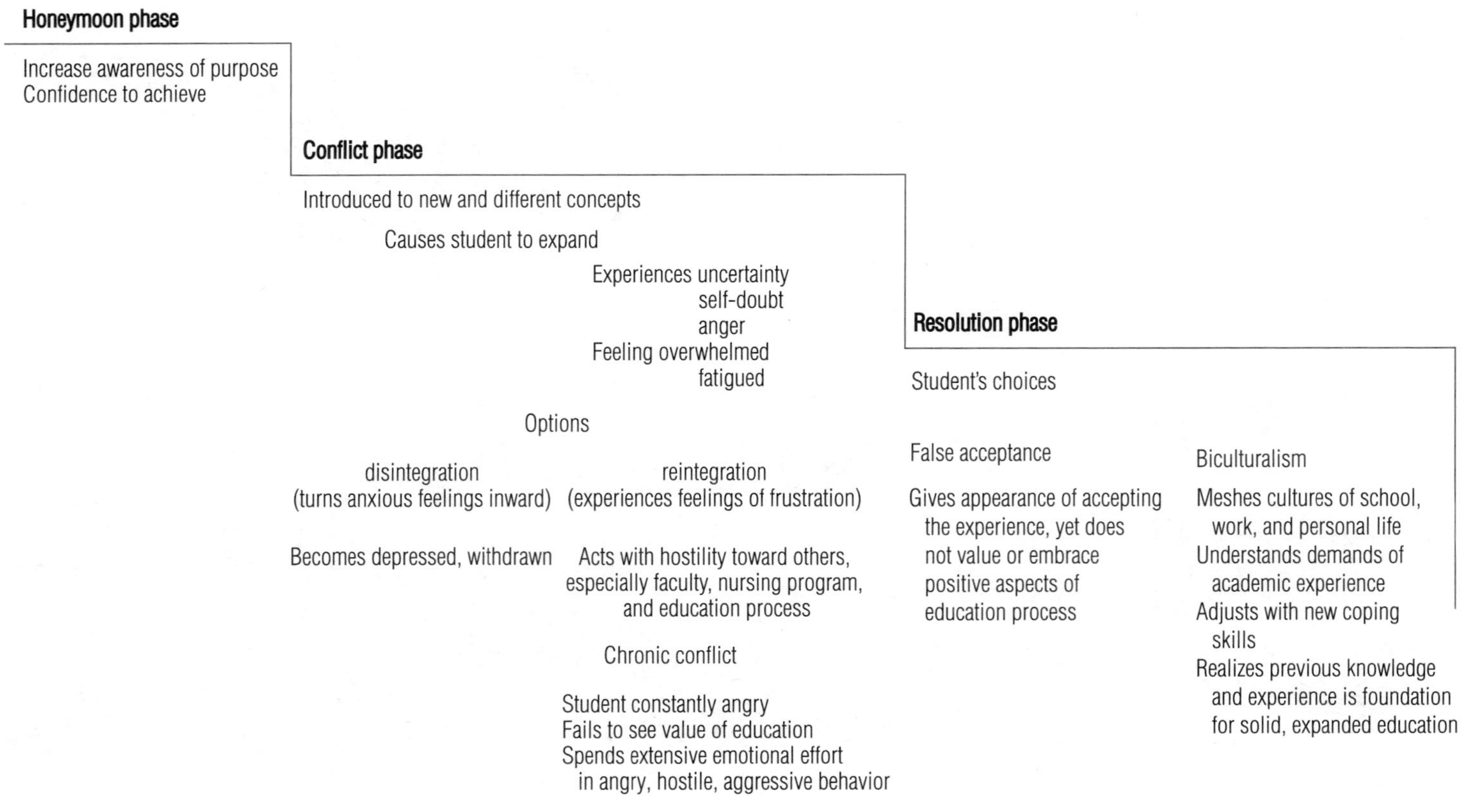

Honeymoon phase

Increase awareness of purpose
Confidence to achieve

Conflict phase

Introduced to new and different concepts

Causes student to expand

Experiences uncertainty
self-doubt
anger

Feeling overwhelmed
fatigued

Options

disintegration   reintegration
(turns anxious feelings inward)   (experiences feelings of frustration)

Becomes depressed, withdrawn   Acts with hostility toward others,
                                especially faculty, nursing program,
                                and education process

Chronic conflict

Student constantly angry
Fails to see value of education
Spends extensive emotional effort
in angry, hostile, aggressive behavior

Resolution phase

Student's choices

False acceptance

Gives appearance of accepting
the experience, yet does
not value or embrace
positive aspects of
education process

Biculturalism

Meshes cultures of school,
work, and personal life
Understands demands of
academic experience
Adjusts with new coping
skills
Realizes previous knowledge
and experience is foundation
for solid, expanded education

Figure 1–1 Returning to School Syndrome (Shane, 1983).

The last phase is the **resolution phase.** Some of the stages in this phase are *chronic conflict, false acceptance,* and *biculturalism.* In the chronic conflict stage, the student is constantly angry, failing to see the value of the education process. She spends extensive emotional effort in angry, hostile, aggressive behavior. In false acceptance, the student gives the appearance of accepting and experiencing the educational process yet does not value or embrace the positive aspects of the educational opportunity. In biculturalism, the student meshes more than one culture, such as school and work, or school and personal life. The student begins to understand the demands of the academic experience and adjusts with new coping skills.

You will not necessarily move through these phases in a linear manner but may move in and out of each phase at different times. Understanding these phases can give you insight as various feelings and emotions arise during the educational experience. You can apply this knowledge to your personal life and learn positive coping skills as you feel these emotions surfacing.

COPING SKILLS

Know that those who have gone before you have also felt the same fears and frustrations. Also, know that they have been rewarded by the same sense of accomplishment you will soon experience.

From Shane's RTSS study, you can become aware of some paths you may want to follow. At first the whole educational experience may seem exciting. Then, as new concepts and more difficult material are presented, realize that you have a choice in your response to the educational experience. Recognizing that you have a choice is gaining insight into ways of coping with life situations. A coping skill is choosing a new way to solve a problem. At times you may feel overwhelmed and uncertain. Fatigue will set in. These feelings are not new to students in education. Rather than *choosing* to feel overwhelmed and anxious, recall your goals, think positive thoughts, spend time with friends who are upbeat, share your feelings with a friend, and know that using some of the study and coping methods presented in this chapter will help sustain you through these times. Rather than striking out at faculty or classmates, realize they may be struggling too, and try to encourage them. Resolve to learn new coping skills to juggle the different responsibilities of home, school, and work. Be open to new nursing concepts and experiences. Compare new concepts with previously learned concepts. By doing this, the educational experience will be a valuable growth experience.

Develop a sense of humor. Appropriate humor and laughter can relieve stressful times when you are caring for clients. Reading comic strips, joke books, and good jokes from Internet friends can develop your sense of humor. If you learn not to take life so seriously and to laugh at your own mistakes, you will release a lot of stress. Some doctors say a good belly laugh a day is good medicine. Laughter definitely gives you a more positive outlook on any situation.

Taking a few minutes to play a simple game with your family also relieves stress. Throwing a Frisbee or playing Yahtzee or other games breaks the monotony of the daily routine. Playing games and laughing with your family offer great opportunities for bonding and many future positive memories.

Playing simple games with a pet also relieves the day's frustration and provides a break in a hectic schedule. Emotionally bonding with a pet provides warmth and security.

DEVELOPING BASIC SKILLS

The nursing environment is constantly changing. Nurses need a variety of new skills to be successful in the work environment. Computer skills are a must. Many doctors' offices are going paperless and using computers only. There may be a computer in the exam room that the doctor and nurse use to record the client's concerns and assessment as the client relates his or her symptoms to them. On clinical units nurses are recording nursing notes on the computer; ordering medications, supplies, and equipment; and obtaining medications from computer-accessed supplies. If you are uncertain about your computer skills, a basic computer course may make for a smoother transition into nursing education.

Basic math and/or algebra are often required in associate degree curricula. Even though many medications are dispensed in unit dose, math skills are still needed to obtain the correct medication dose. If your math skills need a boost, take a math refresher course so you will be ready for the algebra course (see Appendix D). Math and algebra courses also broaden people intellectually and improve critical thinking skills.

An English course is also often required when going for an associate degree. It is important for a nurse to have solid basic English grammar skills. Misspelling words and using poor grammar taint the nursing profession's image. They can also cause legal issues if the wrong subject is referred to in a sentence or if syntax is inaccurate. In administration, nurses may have to write memos and important documents or apply for grants. Good writing skills are needed for these tasks. Therefore, it is important for a nurse to learn basic rules of English grammar and spell correctly.

CRITICAL THINKING ACTIVITIES

1. What phase of the RTSS describes your present feelings?

   _____

   _____

   _____

2. How can you prevent or cope with the conflict phase of the RTSS?

   _____

   _____

   _____

3. What will help you move into the biculturalism stage of the resolution phase of the RTSS?

   _____

   _____

   _____

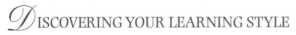

$\mathscr{D}$ISCOVERING YOUR LEARNING STYLE

Your particular learning style is the unique way you perceive information, process it, and then relate the information to others.

As you discover your particular **learning style,** your scope of learning is broadened. You will be able to understand how learning occurs and why it is easier to learn in some classes than in other classes, or the reason that taking a class on-line may appeal to you. You will also be able to understand the rationale of some professors' teaching methods. Discovering your particular learning style will allow you to adapt and learn more effectively.

Anthony Gregorc (1982) describes four learning styles: concrete sequential (CS), concrete random (CR), abstract sequential (AS), and abstract random (AR). He believes one's learning style also determines one's preferred study method (Gregorc & Butler, 1984). Therefore, by determining your learning style, you will learn effective studying methods. Gregorc has also applied learning styles to personality traits and to behaviors in the work environment. By studying learning styles, you will gain insight into your own behavior and the behavior of those with whom you work.

Each of Gregorc's four learning styles is described in the next few paragraphs. Try to identify which one is most like your preferred learning style, and see if the characteristics of that style match your personal characteristics and preferences. By using the study methods listed under the learning style, you will find learning much easier. For example, if your style suggests that you learn best in an environment without distractions, try to find a quiet place to make the most of your study time.

People with a **concrete sequential (CS)** learning style are practical, organized, and structured. The person with a dominant CS style is calm, collected, precise, and strives for perfection. A person scoring high in the CS style works step-by-step, following specific instructions until a project is completed (Gregorc, 1982). Concrete sequential learners prefer a structured, orderly presentation; step-by-step directions; and time for a hands-on experience. They do not tolerate environmental distractions (Gregorc & Ward, 1977). To retain information, the CS learner memorizes or drills. Study method preferences of the CS learner are using workbooks and lab manuals, programmed instruction, computer-aided instruction, organized field trips, demonstration teaching, direct application problems, assembly kits, and hands-on opportunities.

Individuals with a dominant **concrete random (CR)** learning style are creative, independent, and curious. They tend to make quick, impulsive, intuitive decisions. In the workplace, they are the ideas people who do not want to be fenced in but want to be free to express themselves. Their curiosity and competitiveness rarely allow them to accept another's word as fact; instead, the fact must be proven by personal trial and error (Gregorc, 1982). Such people work well on an individual basis and do not respond well to assistance from a teacher in their learning pursuits (Gregorc & Ward, 1977). A person with dominant CR prefers independent study, computer games, open-ended problem solving, simulations, supplemental reading assignments, interactive video, and short lectures with the opportunity to try new methods (Gregorc & Butler, 1984).

Abstract sequential (AS) learners prefer abstract ideas and pictures. Individuals with AS styles may appear flighty or absent-minded, but they love to gather facts, find answers, and debate issues extensively. They are often respected for their intellectual ability. This factor, along with their ability to make long-term plans, leads them into higher education (Gregorc, 1982). Abstract sequential learners prefer lectures, textbooks, supplemental readings, audiotapes, guided individual study, and audiovisual aids, such as videotapes and slide tapes (Gregorc & Butler, 1984). They prefer few environmental distractions (Gregorc & Ward, 1977).

Abstract random (AR) learners are sensitive and flexible. Their approach to the world is based on intuition, emotions, and gut feelings. They are often viewed as daydreamers. Abstract random learners experience the entire learning environment through their emotions (Gregorc, 1982). They prefer to receive information in an unstructured manner and then assimilate the material by reflecting on it (Gregorc & Ward, 1977). They want to belong to the group, and they work well with others, especially in a noncompetitive environment. People with dominant AR style prefer group discussion and enjoy studying with background music. Abstract random learners prefer television, movies, short lectures with questions and answers, guided imagery, and contemplative assignments (Gregorc & Butler, 1984).

A person's cognitive style (the way one processes information) is not limited to learning situations but actually is responsible for one's personality. The behavior patterns evidenced by individual cognitive style have much in common with behavior patterns known as learning style, decision-making style, and social style.

Making Learning Style Adjustments

If the classroom style does not match the student's learning style, the student can still adjust to the classroom mode. Because the student knows how she learns best or her preferred learning style, she can attempt to adjust to the presented style and then make personal adjustments by learning the difficult concepts in her preferred style. For example, if an AR learner is in a class that is presented in a CS manner—using workbooks, computer-aided instruction, and demonstrations—the learner can obtain videos from the library to review concepts, meet with other students to discuss concepts presented in class, or ask questions in class to have the needed personal interaction. This will help the student begin to adapt to styles that are not the preferred style and assist in learning the needed information.

If a student knows her preferred learning style, she also has a preferred study method. The student can use that information to obtain the material needed to assist in the learning process.

Communicating Learning Style to Faculty

There are several learning style assessment tools, such as Anthony Gregorc, Gregorc Style Delineator: A Self-Assessment Instrument for Adults (http://www.Gregorc.com); Dave Kolb (1984), Learning Style Inventory; Peter Honey, Learning Style Questionnaire; and Neil Fleming, VARK: A Guide to Learning Styles (http://www.vark-learn.com). A student can share her personal learning style with the professor and discuss learning style concepts with faculty members. By working together, faculty and student can grow and assist each other in providing a mutually effective learning environment whether that environment is a traditional classroom, on-line, or another distant learning method.

Ideally, faculty members use a variety of methods in presenting information to a class. A student who finds certain concepts difficult can ask the faculty member where those concepts can be found in a different medium. On-line courses that have an interactive option built in can assist some learners.

If the faculty member assists in the student's learning and the student takes personal responsibility for learning, a productive, challenging environment can be created that will hurtle many learning obstacles. Utilizing learning style concepts and providing varied learning methods impact the learning environment in a dramatic way.

CRITICAL THINKING ACTIVITY

1. What is your personal learning style according to the description of each learning style presented in the text? Within that learning style, what are your own best study methods? You may want to complete a learning style inventory, either on-line or by obtaining a learning style assessment tool.

_____

_____

_____

2. Knowing your personal learning style and other learning styles, identify ways you can adapt to a classroom setting in which your personal learning style is not the dominant presentation.

_____

_____

_____

3. How could a person's learning style affect her personality? How could learning style affect a person's work ethic?

_____

_____

_____

TIME MANAGEMENT

Often we vacillate between the feelings expressed in two phrases: "Where has the time gone?" and "Will this time never end?" We all have the same amount of time, but some people use time more effectively and accomplish more than others. Time can either control us, or we can control time by learning to manage activities within an allotted time frame. If we view time as a stopwatch, it controls us. However, we profit if we view time as a continuous growth opportunity to effectively organize activities. That, in a nutshell, is **time management**: effectively prioritizing and organizing responsibilities and activities within a set time frame.

As a returning student, you will consider time a precious commodity. Often academic tasks take twice as long as expected. The juggling of all your roles and responsibilities may seem overwhelming at times. Therefore, a segment of unexpected time is a gift. That is the reason daily judicious prioritizing and organizing of activities is vital.

The academic semester schedule contains monthly, weekly, and daily time segments. At the beginning of each semester, review each course syllabus and record on a monthly calendar project due dates, exam dates, presentation dates, and any special assignment dates for all classes. Also record personal items such as birthdays, ball games, your work schedule, date nights or times with spouse or children, exercise time, and special personal events. Review this for conflicts and possible overload, and adjust the schedule as needed. It is important to maintain this habit, and as each new commitment arises, record it on the monthly calendar. Committing the plan to a written schedule provides direction and a visual reminder.

Some people prefer to break the monthly calendar into weekly or daily calendars. The monthly calendar gives the long-term view, the weekly calendar gives a short-term view offering an opportunity for needed adjustments in preventing a crisis or scheduling conflicts, and the daily view assists with prioritization of activities. By viewing the monthly calendar, you can get an early start on assignments and complete them before their due dates. This decreases physical and emotional stress. Purchasing a computer program that automatically transfers monthly listings to weekly- or daily-planning pages may be very helpful.

One of the best ways to effectively manage responsibilities and time is to complete a daily time plan (see Table 1–1). To make this time plan effective, combine it with a "to do" list. List all items that need completing. The list may seem overwhelming at first, but when you divide it into segments, it will begin to look manageable. Once you have completed the "to do" list, prioritize the items. One way to do this is to number the tasks—for instance, 1 to 10. Another way is to prioritize the items as A (must be done today), B (good if done today), or C (not necessary to do today). Then place all 1 through 5 or A items in the time frames of your daily planner. The time frames should be small segments of time—15 minutes, 30 minutes, or 60 minutes. Experiment with this to see what time segments are most appropriate for you (see Table 1–2 for an example using 30-minute segments). You can make a personal day planner on a computer or purchase one at an office supplies store or campus bookstore.

Table 1–1 Sample daily planner

Done	Time	Schedule	"To do" list	Priority
	7:00			
	7:30			
	8:00			
	8:30			
	9:00			
	9:30			
	10:00			
	10:30			
	11:00			
	11:30			
	12:00			
	12:30			
	1:00			
	1:30			
	2:00			
	2:30			
	3:00			
	3:30			
	4:00			
	4:30			
	5:00			
	5:30			
	6:00			
	6:30			
	7:00			
	7:30			
	8:00			
	8:30			
	9:00			
	9:30			
	10:00			
			Phone calls to make	

Table 1–2 Completed sample daily planner

Done	Time	Schedule	"To do" list	Priority
	7:00		Complete care plan for clinical	B
	7:30		Prep for pharmacology class	A
	8:00	Drop car at repair shop	Buy paint for house	C
	8:30	Study for geriatric nursing exam	Physical therapy on arm	A
	9:00		Pay electric bill	C
	9:30		Drop car at repair shop	A
	10:00	Call Brad's teacher	Get money at bank	B
	10:30		Call Linda	B
	11:00	Prep for pharmacology class	Study for geriatric nursing exam	A
	11:30		Schedule parent-teacher conference	A
	12:00		Mow yard	C
	12:30	Lunch		
	1:00	Pharmacology class		
	1:30			
	2:00			
	2:30			
	3:00			
	3:30			
	4:00			
	4:30	Pick up car at repair shop		
	5:00	Physical therapy on arm		
	5:30			
	6:00	Geriatric nursing class		
	6:30			
	7:00			
	7:30			
	8:00			
	8:30			
	9:00			
	9:30			
	10:00			
			Phone calls to make	
			Call Linda	

At the end of each day, marking off completed items gives a sense of satisfaction. Once you have done that, review the "to do" list again and reorganize the next day. Some items that were not completed may drop off the "to do" list if they have lost their importance. It is best to complete this task at the end of each day, when items that need completing are still fresh in your mind. This way, you can start the next day with purpose, without letting less pressing activities take control of valuable time. Some of you may prefer to prioritize items in the morning when you feel fresh, however. Experiment with different times of the day for completing this activity and see what works best.

STUDY STRATEGIES

By now you may already have developed study methods that work well for you. A review of some survival study skills follows.

Time-Saving Tips

The first priority in being a successful student is to plan time effectively and be as organized as possible.

One way to plan your time effectively and be organized is to use a daily planner to record all assignments, test dates, paper due dates, and study time. Set aside a specific area in your home, at school, or at the library to study. Keep your study area neat and organized. Have a place to file old papers and assignments. Keep separate folders or filing cartons for each class to assist in quickly finding specific papers without sorting through all of them. Use five-minute time segments to make phone calls, contact a classmate to clarify a question or assignment, or review notes. Because most computer paper and assignment papers are 8 1/2 x 11 inches, purchase a 9 x 12–inch zippered notebook to hold your monthly, weekly, and daily planners, phone numbers, and articles or homework that you can work on while waiting in an office or to meet a family member or friend. Accomplish two tasks at once, such as talking on the phone and folding clothes or feeding a pet. Developing effective planning and organizational skills as a student will pay dividends as a nurse.

Class Preparation

Prepare for each week's assignment before class so you glean more from the class content and are ready to participate. Also, advance preparation will allow you to review material for exams, and not study it for the first time just before an exam. It will also prevent the last-minute rush to complete assignments at the end of the semester, which leads to stress.

Effective Note Taking

Learn to take good notes. Devise personal abbreviations for frequently used words. Write phrases, not complete sentences. If you find note taking difficult, outline your reading assignments and then add to or highlight the class members' or instructor's input. The use of a tape recorder in class frees you from the stress of having to write down all the information. You can review the recorded material after class to fill in any gaps in your notes. You can also take notes on a laptop computer. Some faculty members prefer that students request permission prior to using a laptop or tape recorder in class. Review your notes after class while the material is fresh in your mind to cement the information and complete fragmented notes.

Some classes may not have a lecture, note-taking format. Instead, the professor may prefer discussion, presentations, case study review, and other creative educational methods. These offer opportunities for students to adjust to a different type of learning environment. More learning styles are addressed when faculty vary their presentation methods.

Study Time

Set aside study time and inform friends and family of the designated time to prevent interruptions. Let the telephone answering machine record messages during this time so your concentration on study material is not interrupted. Use the designated study time to study; do not allow other activities to fill this scheduled time. The general rule is that a student should spend two to three hours studying for every hour spent in the classroom. The amount of time needed for studying will vary depending on your previous knowledge base of class content. Schedule breaks to prevent sluggishness. If you become drowsy, stand up and move; munch on carrots, celery, or apples; or take a short power nap.

Paper Writing

When writing papers, ask your professor for specific information regarding her expectations for the paper, such as general content, format, inclusion of articles or other references, and specific information to be included. Obtain a copy of the required style guidelines for use at home; APA (American Psychological Association) and MLA (Modern Language Association) are the most frequently required. The APA has a formatting supplement in an electronic version.

Start work early on papers and projects so library personnel can obtain articles, computer information, and books as you need them when writing the paper or completing the project. Begin your own computer searches early so the articles will be available when you need them. Complete the paper early and put it aside for a day, then review it for content change or other needed revisions. Working ahead of schedule decreases stress.

Exam Preparation

Ask your professor as much as possible about exams such as type (multiple choice, true–false, matching, essay); length (timed exam, whole class period); and items you need to bring (calculator, number 2 pencil, book for open-book quiz, or one-page notes if allowed). This information will make your study time more effective because you would prepare differently for each type of exam. Some students find study groups effective to review class material, quiz one another on content, and discuss concepts. Use study groups effectively. Do not substitute personal study time for group study. Study the material first so that you are prepared to contribute to and benefit from the study group. Cramming leads to insecurity when taking exams. Adequate preparation; materials comprehension; and a positive, self-confident attitude decrease test anxiety and lead to test-taking success.

Before beginning the exam, jot down—on the answer sheet or exam paper—rhymes or information that will assist you in recalling information. Ask the professor for clarification if you do not understand the exam material. Pace yourself throughout the exam so that you will have time to complete it.

Grade Games

Some students get caught up in an intense concern and competition for grades that leads to a mental battle for self-esteem. This allows the grade to determine their identity and self-worth. The focus of learning becomes the grade rather than acquiring meaningful information for present and future application. But grades do not always represent the time or energy put into the project. And a grade less than A does not diminish one's identity or self-worth.

CRITICAL THINKING ACTIVITY

1. Review the study strategies and choose two or three methods that you have not used in the past but would like to incorporate into your study skills this semester. Write them down and describe how you will integrate the strategies into your schedule.

_____

_____

_____

_____

_____

$\mathscr{B}$ALANCING HOME, WORK, AND SCHOOL

Chenevert (1997) said the "difference between a goal and a dream is a workable plan" (p. 135). By returning to school for an associate degree, you have set a goal. Now you need to establish plans for attaining your goal that include financial assistance, academic achievement, personal time, and mapped time frames to meet the goal.

In a study of older adults returning to school, Scala (1996) found that students stopped attending classes because of health problems and lack of time for school. In returning to school, a nurse takes on a new role, that of student. Time and energy for each life role (parent, family member, nurse, friend, student, home care provider, employee) come from a finite source. Some students return to school with the "superman complex," thinking that nurses are invincible and can do all things and be all things to all people. Some students attempt to work forty-plus hours a week and still take a full course load. In the process, their health fails and/or their grades suffer. Failure to review and revise personal schedules and work commitments often leads to health issues and lack of study time. Adequate planning can decrease the number of conflicts you encounter in your educational venture.

At various times throughout the educational endeavor, you will experience role strain. This may cause frustration and self-questioning. Explore these feelings with family members, friends, and a school adviser/professor.

Family support is essential when pursuing an associate degree. Your partner and family members may not realize the demands or pressures of school. Communicating the demands and expectations of courses and professors can help your family understand the new pressures on you. Role reversals and delegation of household chores may be helpful during this time. Show family members and friends that their assistance is valued. Perfection is not the name of the game. Clothes do not have to be folded with all corners lined up. Simple meals prepared by children are a luxury. A basic cleaning will do. Pay to have the lawn mowed. If a child or friend is computer literate and can assist with a project, encourage and prize the help. If a friend offers to carpool or baby-sit, accept the assistance. Helping you gives your family and friends a sense of contributing to the project. Therefore, when you finally receive your degree, in essence, your entire family and significant others receive the degree.

Working while going to school can be a stressor or a refreshing outlet. If you are working, discuss a schedule with your supervisor that will accommodate study time, class time, and personal time. Some institutions and companies offer students tuition reimbursement. Working only on weekends may offer more pay along with the freedom to study and spend some leisure time with friends or family during the weekdays.

When students are juggling so many schedules, their physical, emotional, nutritional, and spiritual lives are often neglected. Neglecting social contacts, physical exercise, and spiritual needs can lead to boredom and depression. Have regular contact with a friend over a cup of coffee, in the gym, or at a movie. Exercising three to four times weekly helps maintain a positive attitude and keeps you physically fit. Find an activity you enjoy and participate in it regularly. There are so many good activities to chose, such as walking, biking, racquetball, tennis, and golf. Exercising with friends is an added bonus because it can meet a physical and social need. Maintaining a well-balanced, low-fat diet also aids physical stamina and fitness. Engaging in regular spiritual renewal through worship, prayer, meditation, or study groups meets the spiritual needs that keep us whole.

CRITICAL THINKING ACTIVITY

1. Now that you have completed the monthly, weekly, and daily planners, review the section on balancing home, work, and school and make appropriate adjustments in your schedule. Discuss the planners and adjustments with family, fellow students, or your faculty adviser. It is best to make these adjustments at the beginning of the semester instead of halfway through the semester. How can you put some of these ideas into daily practice?

_____

_____

_____

$\mathcal{S}$UMMARY

Determining personal learning style produces more effective personal study habits and an increased understanding of others' behaviors and learning needs. The stresses of returning to school for an associate degree can be eased as a student develops effective time management skills and study skills and strikes a balance among home, work, and school responsibilities.

Students who return to school for associate degrees often experience a variety of feelings. It is important to understand the RTSS phases to deflect unneeded emotions and take corrective coping actions.

*C*HAPTER REFLECTIONS

1. Refer back to the scenario at the beginning of this chapter. After reading the chapter, what changes do you think Megan may need to make to achieve her educational goals?

2. Do you have trouble managing your time on a daily basis to meet your responsibilities?

3. Identify your learning style and the study skills that will assist you to be successful.

4. Do you have a support network to turn to for assistance?

5. What strategies suggested in this chapter could you apply to your life?

6. How do you feel your personal attitude can influence your educational experience?

REFERENCES

Chenevert, M. (1997). *PRO-Nurse handbook* (3rd ed.). St. Louis: Mosby.

Ezarik, M. (2001). Be a real survivor. *Career World, 30*(2), 6–10.

Green, J. (1996, April 8). LPN-to-RN training: A boon for small hospitals? *AHA News, 32*(14), 5–11.

Gregorc, A. (1982). *An adult's guide to style.* Columbia, CT: Gregorc Associates.

Gregorc, A., & Butler, K. (1984). Learning is a matter of style. *Vocational Education, 4,* 27–29.

Gregorc, A., & Ward, H. B. (1977). Implications for learning and teaching: A new definition for individual. *NASSP Bulletin,* 20–26.

Scala, M. (1996). Going back to school: Participation motives and experience of older adults in an undergraduate program. *Educational Gerontology, 22*(8), 747–774.

Shane, D. (1983). *Returning to school: A guide for nurses.* Englewood Cliffs, NJ: Prentice Hall.

SUGGESTED RESOURCES

Brew, C. (2002). Kolb's learning style instrument: Sensitive to gender. *Educational and Psychological Measurement, 62*(2), 373–390.

Delahoussaye, M. (2002). The perfect learner: An expert debate on learning styles. *Training, 39*(5), 28–36.

Fleming, N. (2001). VARK: A guide to learning styles. http://www.vark learning.com

Gregorc, A. (1985). *Gregorc style delineator: A self-assessment instrument for adults.* Columbia, CT: Gregorc Associates.

Honey, P., & Mumford, A. (1992). *The manual of learning styles.* Maidenhead, Berkshire: Peter Honey Publications.

Kearney, R. (2001). *Advancing your career: Concepts of professional nursing.* Philadelphia: F.A. Davis Company.

Kolb, D. (1984). *Experiential learning: Experience as the source of learning and development.* Englewood Cliffs, NJ: Prentice Hall.

Reese, S. (2002). Understanding our differences. *Techniques, 77*(1), 20–23.

$\mathscr{C}$hapter 2
Role Transition

▼ ▼ ▼ ▼ ▼ ▼ ▼

$\mathscr{L}$EARNING OBJECTIVES

By the end of this chapter, you should be able to:

1. Define the term *role*.
2. Define the nurse's role.
3. Explain the components of the nurse's role.
4. Discuss the transition process from LPN to RN.
5. Discuss the socialization process in becoming an RN.
6. Explain the steps in the change process.
7. Identify ways to use the change process effectively in transitioning from LPN to RN.

$\mathscr{K}$EY TERMS

Advocate

Change agent

Change process

Collaborator

Communicator

Counselor

Educator

Entrepreneur

Leader

Mentor

Researcher

Role

Role conflict

Role model

Role socialization

Role transition

*S*CENARIO

Jefferson is entering the transitions class for licensed practical nurses (LPNs) in an associate degree in nursing (ASN) program at a local university. He feels the transitions class is not really necessary because he has been dealing with transitions his entire life. His nursing career began in high school when he worked as a nursing assistant in a nursing home. After high school he became a qualified medical assistant (QMA) and, eventually, an LPN. So, here he is today working on his associate degree . . . what is one more step up the nursing ladder? Jefferson feels that making a bed is making a bed . . . passing medication is passing medication . . . nursing is nursing! He says, "What's the big deal? I'm already doing everything the RNs are doing!"

*T*HINK ABOUT IT

1. How did Jefferson's responsibilities change for each of his roles, from QMA to LPN and, finally, RN? Do you think his employer or other members of the health care team had higher expectations as he climbed the nursing ladder?

2. Do changes in roles, such as moving from LPN to RN, affect the attitudes of co-workers toward you and what you are doing?

3. As you move toward your RN role, how do you feel about the other nursing positions (QMA, LPN, etc.)? Do people in these positions have value on the health care team, or should they be following in your footsteps in education?

*I*NTRODUCTION

You have just embarked on a new adventure that will require an adjustment in your professional role. In the previous chapter we discussed strategies to assist you as you make the transition to the student role. In this chapter we will focus on the transition and socialization process needed in making the change from LPN to RN, and the role conflicts you may encounter in the transition. We will define the nursing role and look at the components of that role. We will also explore the change process in making the transition from LPN to RN. By the end of the chapter you will have information to assist you in becoming an RN.

$\mathscr{T}$YPES OF ROLE

---

*A **role** is a set of expectations society assumes a person in a certain position or occupation will perform.*

A **role** is a set of expectations society assumes a person in a certain position or occupation will perform. Each of us assumes various roles in the course of a day. Some of these roles may be parent, partner, friend, counselor, chauffeur, teacher, chef, and nurse. As a nurse completes his daily personal and professional responsibilities, he assumes many roles to complete the work effectively.

What changes are needed to become an RN?

Some LPN students may enter nursing education thinking their nursing role will not change once they become an RN. They believe they will still use the clinical skills they have been using as an LPN. Some clinical duties *will* be the same, and the LPN often performs them with expertise. So, what changes are needed to become an RN?

In becoming an RN, the LPN student will change, or make a role transition, in personal identity and role function (Amos, 2001). One of the main changes that will occur is performance of the same clinical skills with improved and refined critical thinking. Rather than doing a routine procedure, an LPN-RN student will learn to analyze diagnostic test results, analyze the client's overall condition, and evaluate whether the procedure should be done on the client. He will then accept the responsibility of using his own critical thinking skills to determine whether the client's condition may be jeopardized by the procedure. Critical thinking skills are continually refined throughout the education experience. The refinement and application of critical thinking is part of transitioning into the role of RN.

CRITICAL THINKING ACTIVITY

1. What role changes do you anticipate occurring in your life in the next two years?

   _____

   _____

   _____

2. Think of three specific ways your professional role will change by becoming an RN.

   _____

   _____

   _____

$\mathcal{R}$OLE COMPONENTS

The nurse's roles include advocate, counselor, researcher, mentor, collaborator, change agent, educator, entrepreneur, role model, leader, and communicator.

Some of the roles society may place on a nurse are competent worker, organized care provider, knowledgeable caregiver, caring person, and hard worker. In fact, the nurse's roles include advocate, counselor, researcher, mentor, collaborator, change agent, educator, entrepreneur, role model, leader, and communicator (Figure 2–1). We will discuss these role responsibilities to gain a better understanding of the RN's role.

Advocate

An **advocate** speaks for or acts on behalf of another person. At times, this is the role of the nurse. The client may need the nurse to speak to a doctor on his behalf. It is the duty of the nurse to act on behalf of the client. A nurse may ask a physician to repeat an explanation of a scheduled procedure to a nonassertive client. A nurse may stand up for a client's right to refuse a procedure. "Because of nursing's presence, patient and family are never alone, never left uncared for or uninformed, and never left without an advocate" (Dickenson-Hazard, 2000, p. 8).

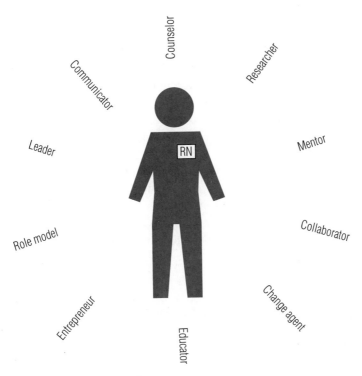

Figure 2–1 Nurses' roles.

Counselor

A nurse is a **counselor** when he listens to a client and uses therapeutic communication to assist the client in making a choice that determines his health outcome. For example, a nurse as a counselor may lend an ear to a client who is debating two or more choices. It is important for the nurse to explain, define, and review the client's options. The final decision, however, always remains with the client. A client may be deciding, for instance, whether to proceed with chemotherapy treatment at a local hospital or seek other treatment options at the Mayo Clinic. The nurse answers questions and reviews options with the client, but the treatment decision ultimately lies with the client.

The RN's education has prepared him to identify a client's emotional status. The RN identifies the client's anxiety level, assesses the client's coping skills, and determines the client's defense mechanisms. This knowledge will assist in counseling the client.

Researcher

A nurse is faced with many scientific problems to solve or questions to answer each day. What is the best way to treat pressure sores? Is a certain type of dressing more absorbent than another, and, if it is, how does that affect the client's healing process? Is medication X more effective for the client than medication Y? What are the benefits and side effects of each? In participating in clinical research on scientific questions such as these, the RN functions as a **researcher**. The goal of nursing research is to improve the quality of client nursing care. An RN develops research questions, collects data for research, values research results, and applies research findings to practice. A master's- or doctorate-credentialed RN is usually the nurse who conducts research. However, all RNs can be involved in collecting data for research and in initiating nursing research questions.

Mentor

Webster's New World Dictionary and Thesaurus defines **mentor** as "a wise, loyal adviser." As a mentor, the nurse is a wise adviser to a new graduate or new employee and is loyal to that individual by assisting him with unit procedures and policies, explaining unit equipment, and walking alongside the new nurse, easing his adjustment to the unit in every possible way.

Sometimes a mentor is called a *nurse preceptor*. A new nurse is assigned to another nurse, a preceptor, who assists the new nurse as he transitions onto the unit. The preceptor fulfills the role of a confidant, allowing the new nurse to ask questions in a safe, supportive environment so that the nurse can smoothly adapt to the work environment and the role of nurse. This type of program often enhances recruitment and retention of nurses. An RN fulfills the role of a mentor or preceptor. Even if the mentor/preceptor role is not part of a formal program, it is important that every RN assume the mentor role when a new nurse comes into the work environment.

Collaborator

The nurse **collaborator** interacts with the personnel of several departments to coordinate the client's care. The client may be referred to physical therapy, occupational therapy, radiology, surgery, and social services. The nurse skillfully schedules and communicates the client's needs to each of these departments and fulfills the role of collaborator. An RN assumes the role of collaborator by meeting with multidisciplinary personnel to achieve the client's goal of maximum health and by meeting with family members to plan care with the client. In completing these tasks, the RN may delegate responsibilities to other nurses and then follow up on the delegated tasks.

Change Agent

In our present health care delivery system, changes occur on a daily basis. Often these changes are brought about by nurses or with the nurse's input. The nurse needs to be familiar with the change process and to become a vital **change agent**. The "idea person" is an essential asset to the nursing unit and nursing in general. Not only does the nurse need to be creative, but he also needs to possess the personal and communication skills to persuade others that change is needed and to bring about the needed change as smoothly as possible. Some units function more smoothly when nurses work 12-hour shifts or if shift flexibility is provided. The nurse can be a vital change agent to persuade a facility's administration and the nursing staff to try the idea of flexible shift scheduling. The RN can be a dynamic change agent by writing proposals, making appointments with administrators and sharing their ideas, actively participating in staff meetings, and becoming an active committee member.

Not only are nurses change agents within the health care system, but they also can play a very effective and influential role in the formation of public policy. They can write legislators and influence politicians regarding legislative bills for home health care and health care in general. Issues that still need resolution are prescription coverage for the elderly, large companies' giving kickbacks to physicians for prescribing their branded drugs rather than encouraging physicians to prescribe generic drugs, and staffing issues in nursing homes and hospitals. RNs become aware of and have the opportunity to get involved in current issues by reading newspapers, listening to or watching local and world news programs, reviewing bill proposals on-line, e-mailing politicians, and participating in professional nursing organizations.

Educator

All nurses perform the role of **educator** on a daily basis with clients as they explain procedures, lab tests, disease processes, and care interventions. Through the education process, an RN is taught critical thinking techniques to meet the emotional needs of clients as procedures and diagnostic tests are explained.

The RN often functions as a staff educator. He reads current literature and shares new knowledge with co-workers. As research is published, he shares the findings with co-workers and applies them to client care. It is important that nurses recognize the role of educator and make learning a lifelong process through attending seminars and local presentations and reading current literature.

Entrepreneur

A nurse may become an **entrepreneur** by venturing into health care businesses. Many are doing so. Nurses willing to take a business challenge and use their professional skills can fill gaps in the health care system. These nurses have expanded the scope of nursing and health care. Nurse entrepreneurs are offering health education, ostomy care, aromatherapy, case management, and counseling services. Recently, three LPNs started an adult day care center in a moderate-sized midwestern U.S. city. Nurse practitioners are starting and managing health clinics.

Health care entrepreneurship is limited only by lack of imagination and initiative.

There are several steps to take to embark on this type of venture. First, the nurse sees a need that is not being met in the present health care system. Second, he completes a market analysis (or hires someone to complete one) to see if the product or service is truly needed in the community. Third, he completes a market test with the product or service, followed by a business trial run. Before becoming an entrepreneur, the nurse must have a solid knowledge of the business world and of government policies addressing the desired business (Hood & Leddy, 2003). Health care entrepreneurship is limited only by lack of imagination and initiative.

Role Model

A nurse may be a **role model**, a professional example for student nurses and new graduates. Nurses can also be role models as they interact with clients, health care team members, and co-workers. A nurse who facilitates a positive, encouraging, supportive work environment can be one of the best role models on the health care team.

Leader

RNs often assume the role of **leader** as they manage client care, hospital units, and clinics. However, leadership can also be demonstrated in decisive decision making and in accepting autonomy, responsibility, and accountability in providing competent care. Dickenson-Hazard (2000) states, "Every nurse is a leader . . . [because] every nurse exercises leading-edge authority to influence the health of those in his or her care." It is important for the LPN-RN student to learn leadership skills.

When an RN assumes leadership responsibilities, sometimes co-workers become jealous and make the job more difficult for him. When co-workers become leaders, a professional nurse supports and encourages the RNs to be successful in their new leadership role.

Communicator

The art of therapeutic communication is taught in nursing education because communication skills are essential for nurses. The nurse as **communicator** uses therapeutic communication to relate information and to explore clients' feelings and thoughts. So often, these skills are forgotten in the rush of daily responsibilities. Yet it is important to communicate in a therapeutic manner with a client.

The techniques of therapeutic communication are also effective in interpersonal communication. It is a joy to see nurses communicate effectively with one another as their communication skills become second nature.

CRITICAL THINKING ACTIVITIES

1. List nurse role components other than those described in the text.

   _____

   _____

   _____

2. How many of the role components described here have you fulfilled as an LPN?

_____

_____

_____

3. What entrepreneurial ventures would you like to undertake if money, life responsibilities, or other issues were not a factor?

_____

_____

_____

4. Give an example of effective communication you witnessed at work or on a clinical site.

_____

_____

_____

5. What political nursing issue would you like to address with a legislator?

_____

_____

_____

6. Choose an RN in a role you find interesting in your community. Shadow the RN for one day and then list the components of his or her role.

_____

_____

_____

$\mathscr{R}$OLE SOCIALIZATION

As you move through the educational process, your clinical nursing skills will expand, you will acquire new critical thinking abilities, and you will internalize a new personal identity.

As you move through the educational process, your clinical nursing skills will expand, you will acquire new critical thinking ability, and you will internalize a new personal identity. Your LPN education is very important and will be utilized in developing this new role. You have chosen to move to a different level in your education and professional status. This involves a process called role socialization. In the role socialization process, personal identity meshes with professional identity. In your case, you have professionally identified with the associate degree nursing role. **Role socialization** is developing an internal attitude toward a profession. When role socialization occurs, you can proudly say, "I am an associate degree nurse." You had this same feeling when you became an LPN, and now you are in the process of assuming a new identity—that of an associate degree nurse. The resocialization process began when you decided to enroll in the associate degree program. During the educational process, you will learn new skills and a new way of thinking and you will have a chance to develop new values toward the nursing profession.

As an adult learner, you have some special expectations and goals for the educational process. Lawler (1991) lists nine principles of adult learning. As you read these nine principles, examine their relevance to your present philosophy of education.

1. Adult learning requires an atmosphere of respect.
2. A cooperative, two-way learning environment is essential to adult education.
3. Adult education builds on the education of the participant.
4. Adult education encourages critical contemplative thinking.
5. Adult education presents situational problems and encourages problem solving.
6. Adult education is pertinent and applicable.
7. Adult education is an active, give and take process with the adult learner taking part in the learning process.
8. Adult education gives power and immeasurable opportunity to the learner.
9. Adult education stimulates the learner to be self-directed and independent.

These nine principles are essential for the LPN-RN student. The LPN comes to the learning environment with a foundation of knowledge and experience to be refined and advanced to the next educational level.

It is important for the LPN to have a voice and be involved in the learning process. One way you can involve yourself in the learning process is to collaborate with staff and faculty members as you are learning new nursing concepts. In the learning environment, seek to find solutions to clinical and client problems. The staff and nursing faculty serve as role models to demonstrate critical thinking skills. Take the opportunity to interact with staff and faculty members to examine and analyze clinical situations.

Your experience as an LPN provides you with confidence, comfort, and a degree of independence in the clinical environment. As you collaborate with staff and faculty members, seek feedback as to ways you can improve your critical thinking skills and clinical performance. This is an opportunity for the LPN to blossom and reach full potential.

During the process of becoming an RN, it is important for the LPN to value past education and, at the same time, meet the challenge of accepting new ideas, improving critical thinking skills, and learning new nursing techniques.

During the process of becoming an RN, it is important for the LPN to value past education and, at the same time, meet the challenge of accepting new ideas, improving critical thinking skills, and learning new nursing techniques. This will be a time of tremendous growth and change.

Hood and Leddy (2003, p. 97) state, "The socialization process involves changes in knowledge, attitudes, values, and skills. These changes can be associated with conflict and strong emotional reactions." The process of acquiring new skills, knowledge, and values may occur several times in your lifetime. Two role socialization transitions that will soon occur in your life are adjusting to the educational process and adapting to the new role of registered nurse. Throwe and Fought (1987) developed a resocialization assessment tool (Table 2–1) that uses Erik Erickson's theory of developmental stages to identify changes that will occur in a nurse's life as he either resists or accepts a new role identity. You can use this tool periodically to evaluate your personal progress in role socialization as you advance through your educational experience and move into your role as an associate degree nurse.

Table 2–1 Resocialization assessment tool

Developmental Task	Role-Resisting Behaviors Observed	Role-Accepting Behaviors Observed
Trust/mistrust		
Learns to trust the worlds of education and work through consistency and repetitive experiences	Physically isolated from peers both in class, clinical Does not initiate interactions with others Responds only if called on	Involved with classmates Readily and quickly forms/joins groups when directed Initiates discussions with others Asks for clarification
Autonomy/doubt		
Begins to develop independence while under supervision	Delays joining groups for unstructured activities Does not contribute easily Forgets or suppresses assignment dates Does not meet target dates Self-conscious about being evaluated by others	Joins groups for unstructured activities (study groups) Shares information with group, prepares for activities Meets target dates Able to interact in the teaching/learning environment Begins to develop independence with guidance
Initiative/guilt		
Can independently identify plan, and implement skills/assignments	Perceives objectives and assignments as not worthwhile Stress-related symptoms increase Has difficulty setting priorities Waits for instructor to initiate priority setting Lacks initiative to deal with conflicts Unaware of available resources	Objectives and assignments take on meaning Applies new skills, content to other work settings Effective in time management Renegotiates deadline extensions when appropriate Takes initiative in resolving conflict situations Aware of and uses available resources

Table 2–1 (continued)

Industry/inferiority

Behavior is dominated by performance of tasks and curiosity—individuals need encouragement to attempt and master skills	Elicits performance rewards and feedback from others	Able to reward self
	Needs direct encouragement especially when performing affective and cognitive skills	Confidence thrives
	Last to volunteer to demonstrate new behaviors	Eager to try out new skills; takes risks
	Seeks rewards by performing old familiar skills rather than those in new dimensions	Volunteers to demonstrate new behaviors
	Demonstrates disengaging behaviors (late, uninterested, resistive to learning opportunities)	Profits from guidance and direction of others
		Applies self beyond family/work setting
		Curiosity channeled through education system

Identity/role confusions

The individual searches for continuity and structure, is concerned with how he/she is accepted by others; how he/she is accepted by self; each individual struggles to shape or formulate own identity	Needs a structured clinical setting to further develop ego identity	Searches for continuity and structure but can adapt to unstructured clinical settings
	Sees old job as ideal and denies need for change	Identifies role models in clinical setting
	Serious about learning (content and clinical) practice	Articulates need for change or for modification of job-related roles and procedures
	Frustrated with nursing as a career choice	Appears to enjoy learning and performing in clinical settings
	Too ideological or overly critical of others	Idealistic about own achievements and progress in educational system

Table 2–1 (continued)

Intimacy/isolation

Seeks to combine his/her identity with other self-selected individuals	Participates as a member but resists group leader role	Volunteers to lead work/study groups
	Does not participate in professional meetings	Participates in professional organizations
	Unsupportive of others' educational advancement	Recruits others and represents school
	Feels no increased esteem in performing new role behaviors	Demonstrates pride in new role behaviors and shares with others in work settings
	Meets minimal requirements and sees instructor only in evaluative role	Seeks out instructor for additional learning, information, and professional growth opportunities
	Resists using newly developed skills, more comfortable with previous level of performance	Values symbols of profession (using assessment tools, RN name tags)
	Avoids giving feedback to agency personnel	Evaluates ability of clinical agencies to facilitate meeting learner objectives
		Provides feedback to agency personnel

Table 2–1 (continued)

Generativity/stagnation

Efforts are made to guide and direct incoming students; assists others	Avoids social interaction and information sharing with incoming students	Guides and directs incoming students
	Provides minimal care, unconcerned about continuity of patient care	Provides quality nursing care to patient, family, and community
	Selects patients with common familiar clinical disorders	Takes calculated risks (questions level of care, seeks multiple learning opportunities, shares level of expertise, elects to test out required elective courses)
	No increased ease of learning or improved test-taking abilities	Demonstrates critical problem-solving skills
	Does not elect to test out of course requirements	Attains mastery of test-taking skills
	Stagnates in same job setting	Self-directed learner
		Demonstrates clinical problem-solving in own work setting
		Uses holistic approach to delivery of health care

Ego integrity/despair

Acceptance of one's own progress, achievement, and goals through realistic self-appraisal	Frustrated with progress and achievement; stagnated in developing new goals	Accepts progress, achievement and goal attainment
	Crisis prone when changing roles	Realistic in self-appraisal
	Self appraisal unrealistic	Resets professional goals (graduate school, participation in continuing education, certification)
	Does not participate in structured educational opportunities	Joins new perspectives on old job by use of critical thinking
	Returns to old job and does not modify role performance	Takes risks (new jobs, different clinical setting, and leadership roles)
	Sees no reward in risk-taking	
	High risk for dissatisfaction with profession	

CRITICAL THINKING ACTIVITIES

1. At what point did you truly identify or become socialized in your role as a new LPN? What were the biggest factors in shaping your professional identity?

    _____

    _____

    _____

2. Describe where you are today in the socialization process as an LPN-RN student.

    _____

    _____

    _____

3. Choose three of the nine principles of adult learning that are most important to you. Explain the significance of these three principles to your present educational process.

    _____

    _____

    _____

ℛOLE TRANSITION

Role transition implies a change in one's role requirements, expectations, and work responsibilities. It also requires an internal change in the way one thinks about or views the new role.

Role transition implies a change in one's role requirements, expectations, and work responsibilities. It also requires an internal change in the way one thinks about or views the new role. As you move through the process of becoming a registered nurse, your job requirements, expectations, and work responsibilities will change. At first you may think that you are performing the same responsibilities. To a degree you are. You still change dressings, administer medications, and assess clients. However, as you progress in the education process, you will perform these duties with more knowledge, critical thinking skills, and nursing judgment. A role transition will be occurring. This will be a process, not an overnight change.

Nicholson and West (1988) describe four stages in work transitions when a company downsizes. These four stages (preparation, encounter, adjustment, and stabilization) also relate to other life transitions (see Figure 2-2).

The preparation stage is mostly concerned with psychological preparedness for the transition that is to occur. When changing roles from LPN to RN, one must psychologically desire to make the change. The LPN examines personal qualities and decides if he possesses the personal mental and emotional abilities needed to become an RN. During this time, the LPN may closely watch RNs to see how they function and what they do. Then, the LPN measures the skills seen against his own abilities.

The encounter phase is the first few days and weeks after the initial psychological decision has been made. During the encounter phase, the LPN makes the necessary contacts to enroll in college, makes financial arrangements, and revises his personal schedule to accommodate class and clinical schedules. The LPN in this stage may experience a feeling of loss or disconnectedness.

In the adjustment stage, one focuses on and establishes a new set of priorities. The LPN may find that previous relationships with co-workers change as he makes the appropriate changes in his work role. Some of these changes will begin occurring during schooling and will continue after the LPN has become an RN, as he takes on the culture of the new RN role. In this stage, the LPN may feel somewhat pulled between two worlds: the world of the previous LPN role, and the world of the RN role.

In the stabilization stage, the LPN takes on the values of the RN role. He makes adjustments and minor changes as needed and enjoys the successes of the new role.

Viewing the transition as a challenging opportunity will help prepare you emotionally and mentally for the growth process.

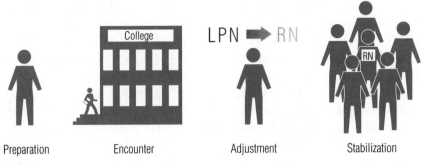

| Preparation | Encounter | Adjustment | Stabilization |

Figure 2–2 Stages in work transition.

Viewing the transition as a challenging opportunity will help prepare you emotionally and mentally for the growth process. The movie *Dead Poet's Society* used a phrase appropriate in transition. It is *carpe diem*, "seize the day." Seize the opportunity this transition offers you. The rewards will be bountiful.

CRITICAL THINKING ACTIVITIES

1. How did you feel when you transitioned into the LPN role? What surprised you the most? What do you wish you had done differently?

   _____

   _____

   _____

2. Identify your present transition phase in becoming an RN.

   _____

   _____

   _____

*R*OLE CONFLICT

Role conflict occurs when a person's role has two or more conflicting or incompatible expectations.

Role conflict occurs when a person's role has two or more conflicting or incompatible expectations. From the individual's perspective, the two role expectations seem to conflict with each other, and therefore, the person experiences a dilemma in trying to assume both roles.

Role conflicts can be intrapersonal or interpersonal. An example of an intrapersonal conflict is a student who needs to study but feels guilty for not spending more time with significant others, or who struggles to meet school responsibilities and other social obligations. Interpersonal conflict occurs when other people's expectations differ or conflict with each other or with one's personal view of the role. An example of an interpersonal conflict is a doctor's requesting a nurse to perform a procedure in a manner contrary to a facility's policy. The nurse would have a role conflict between the doctor's expectations and the employer's expectations.

An LPN who is going for an associate degree in nursing may experience role conflict both emotionally and physically. Emotionally, the LPN may struggle because he is content as an LPN yet he is receiving pressure from an employer to become an RN. The LPN may struggle with knowing, from his perspective, how to perform a clinical skill but needing to relearn certain methods of doing the procedure to successfully pass the procedure in a lab check-off. If an LPN is working while going to school, the LPN may struggle with being able to perform a procedure as an RN student but not while working as an LPN. The role expectations in each of these situations are incompatible, leading to a potential role conflict. As these conflicts build, the person may develop hypertension, peptic ulcers, or other psychosomatic illnesses.

The LPN student can avoid some of these conflicts by prioritizing tasks, using effective communication skills, and appropriately delegating responsibilities. For example, in dealing with the previously stated conflict between doctor and employer expectations, the nurse uses assertive communication skills. He states that his employer has certain expectations of him in completing the procedure, and, therefore, he will not be able to do the procedure as the doctor has requested.

CRITICAL THINKING ACTIVITY

1. Describe a time when you experienced a role conflict.

_____

_____

_____

THE CHANGE PROCESS

Change is a certainty in life. A **change process** is your response to pressures during various life experiences that cause modifications in behavior. The health care system has undergone and is still experiencing the effects of change with facility mergers and the nursing shortage.

Change can occur because of an external force or an internal force. An external force is brought about by a situation outside of ourselves or by something that we cannot control. An internal force arises within ourselves and stems from a personal desire for something different.

We usually adapt more easily to internal forces than to external forces because the motivation for change starts within us and is not done to us.

Kurt Lewin developed the classic change theory in 1951. Since that time, others have modified the change theory but still use the three stages of Lewin's theory: unfreezing, moving, and refreezing (Figure 2–3). Lewin's theory is based on restraining forces and driving forces (Figure 2–4). Restraining forces are the issues in life or in society that resist change, such as fears, perceived threats, values, and relationships. Driving forces are the motivators to change, such as a desire for a different method or operational norm.

The unfreezing phase can be an uncomfortable, restless time as a person senses or is told a change is about to occur. If the person desires the change, there is less uneasiness at this time. During this phase, there is a struggle between the restraining and driving forces as they jockey to resist or change the status quo.

In the moving phase, the person has accepted the change and is setting goals to determine the direction of the change. If the change involves several people, it is important to have all of them involved during this time. Change is easier if everyone feels they have input and that their input is valued.

In refreezing, equilibrium has been established and the change has become the new status quo. The benefits of the change are emphasized during this time.

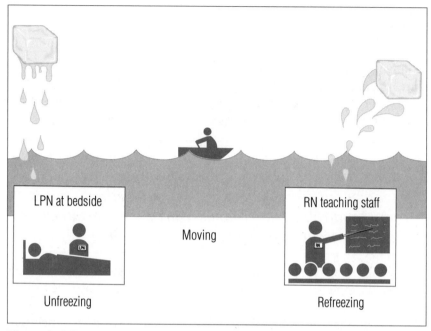

LPN at bedside

Moving

RN teaching staff

Unfreezing

Refreezing

Figure 2–3 Three stages of Lewin's change theory.

An example of the change process is your return to school to become an RN. In the unfreezing stage, you went through a process to decide to return to school. The decision may have been more difficult for some of you than for others. Perhaps you personally made the decision and it affected only you. Or perhaps you made the decision but needed to discuss its ramifications with your family. Perhaps an employer made the decision for you. You may have experienced a time of discomfort or a time of motivation, depending whether the decision was an internal force or an external force. In the moving phase, you had to make goals and plans to accomplish the task of returning to school. In the refreezing phase, your adaptation to student life is (or will be) reinforced and your student role becomes the new status quo. Once you graduate, the change process will occur again as you adapt to the new nursing work environment.

CRITICAL THINKING ACTIVITY

1. Describe a change process in which you have been involved. What was your role? What were the restraining forces? What

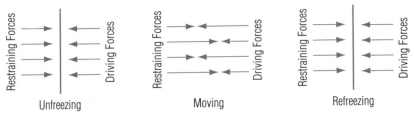

Unfreezing   Moving   Refreezing

Figure 2–4 Restraining forces versus driving forces.

were the driving forces? How were others motivated or mobilized in the moving phase?

_____

_____

_____

_____

_____

ＳUMMARY

When parents take children to a fine-dining restaurant, they expect the children to place their napkin in their lap, use the appropriate fork with the appropriate food, and behave in an approved manner. The children are transitioning into a new socialization process.

To a degree, that dining experience is somewhat like the transition from LPN to RN. The RN's role includes a set of expectations in behavior and analytical thinking that can be broken down into specific functional components. An LPN may have completed certain aspects of these expectations, but in becoming an RN, they will be expanded. A socialization process occurs, and the LPN internalizes the values of an RN and takes on a new identity.

Adults entering an educational experience also have certain expectations. They are self-directed and desire to be an integral part of the educational experience. Faculty members will model critical thinking skills and competence in assessing the client's health status. The LPN will learn the critical thinking skills and clinical expertise needed to function as a competent, decisive, caring nurse.

Transitioning and socialization are change processes. The LPN may experience many interpersonal and intrapersonal emotions and conflicts. He will relearn some nursing procedures, refine his thinking, expand his nursing concepts, and his self-confidence will grow. As the LPN moves through the change process from unfreezing to refreezing, he is equipping himself to move through these steps again and again throughout his nursing career.

$\mathcal{C}$HAPTER REFLECTIONS

1. After reading the chapter, do you feel that you can be an advocate, researcher, mentor, collaborator, and change agent? Were you already doing these things as a nursing assistant, QMA, and/or LPN?

2. Describe the role differences between LPN and RN. Really stop and think about it. What changes can you anticipate as you become an RN?

3. Is this change in your life happening because of an external force or an internal force? Why do you want to become an RN? What stage of Lewin's change theory are you now experiencing?

REFERENCES

Amos, D. (2001). An evaluation of staff nurse role transition. *Nursing Standard, 16*(3), 36–45.

Dickenson-Hazard, N. (2000). Every nurse is a leader. *Nursing, 30*(11), 8–9.

Hood, L., & Leddy, S. (2003). *Leddy and Pepper's Conceptual bases of professional nursing* (5th ed.). Philadelphia: Lippincott Williams & Williams.

Laird, C., & Agnus, M. (2002). *Webster's New World Dictionary and Thesaurus* (2nd ed.). Indianapolis: John Wiley & Sons.

Lawler, P. (1991). *The keys to adult learning: Theory and practical strategies.* Philadelphia: Research for Better Schools.

Lewin, K. (1951). *Field theory in social science.* New York: Harper & Row.

Nicholson, N., & West, M. (1988). *Managerial job change: Men and women in transition.* Cambridge, England: Cambridge University Press.

Throwe, A., & Fought, S. (1987). Landmarks in the socialization process from RN to BSN. *Nurse Educator, 12,* 16–17.

SUGGESTED RESOURCES

Allen, T., Freeman, D., Russell, J., Reizenstein, R., & Rentz, J. (2001). Survivor reactions to organizational downsizing: Does time ease the pain? *Journal of Occupational and Organizational Psychology, 74*(2), 145–164.

Joel, L. (2002). Reflections and projections on nursing. *Nursing Administration Quarterly, 26*(5), 11–17.

Chapter 3
LPN and RN Knowledge and Roles

▼ ▼ ▼ ▼ ▼ ▼ ▼

LEARNING OBJECTIVES

By the end of this chapter, you should be able to:

1. List the LPN's role and responsibilities.
2. List the RN's role and responsibilities.
3. List the associate degree RN's core components and competencies.
4. Evaluate your role and responsibilities as an LPN.
5. Define the differences between LPN and RN roles and responsibilities.

KEY TERMS

Assessment
Caring interventions
Clinical decision making
Collaboration
Communication
Core components and competencies
Learning
LPN responsibilities
LPN roles
Managing care
Professional behaviors
RN responsibilities
RN roles
Teaching

$\mathcal{S}$CENARIO

Kimberly has been an LPN for the last 15 years, and, in that time, she has functioned in many capacities. She was taught many different skills: inserting IVs, caring for central venous lines, blood draws, special dressing changes, and inserting nutritional supplements into feeding tubes of all sizes. She was a very skillful nurse. She also began functioning in a leadership role after being an LPN for just one year, supervising a building of 100 clients, 24 of them in a skilled bed and another 20 with Alzheimer's. She also was responsible for guiding and directing approximately 30 employees at a time. She made their work assignments and coordinated their responsibilities throughout the shift. Kimberly dealt with family concerns and client crises, and she assisted in reaching a solution to problems. When asked why she is returning to school, Kimberly responds, "Hey, I'm already doing everything the RNs are doing. I might as well get the title and pay along with the work."

$\mathcal{T}$HINK ABOUT IT

1. Compare the job descriptions of an LPN and an RN. Are you aware of the Nurse Practice Act for the state in which you practice? Review what you are doing in your current role. Is it within your nurse practice guidelines?

2. Is there a difference between RN and LPN thinking and problem solving? Do you find that an LPN reports to and is guided through difficult situations by an RN mentor?

$\mathcal{I}$NTRODUCTION

At this point you may be asking yourself, So what *is* the difference between the LPN and the RN? In this chapter we will compare and contrast the roles, responsibilities, and knowledge levels of the LPN and the RN. We will examine and candidly discuss similarities and differences between the LPN and the RN. Together, we will gain respect for and learn to value the roles and competencies of both the LPN and the RN.

$\mathcal{N}$ATIONAL NURSING ORGANIZATIONS' DEFINITIONS OF NURSING ROLES

To establish a valid difference between the LPN and the RN, we need to review how national licensing organizations and national nursing organizations define LPNs and RNs. Their defining statements are based on data, research studies, and councils of nurses.

In 1988 Kane and Colton conducted a job analysis of newly licensed LPNs to establish the entry-level practices of LPNs. Using their data, the National Council of State Boards of Nursing (NCSBN) developed the National Council Licensure Examination for Practical Nurses (NCLEX-PN). In 1993, Chornick, Yocom, and Jacobson conducted a job analysis study similar to the previous LPN study to establish the entry-level practices for RNs. From this study, the National Council Licensure Examination for Registered Nurses (NCLEX-RN) was designed. Cognitive abilities tested on both the LPN and the RN exams are *knowledge, comprehension,* and *application.* The main testing difference between the LPN and the RN exams is that the RN exam has an *analysis* component. Knowledge is the facts; for example, What is the kidney bean–shaped organ in the lower back? Comprehension is the understanding of the facts; for example, Describe the function of the kidney. Application is applying facts or putting the facts to use; for example, What could an elevated blood urea nitrogen (BUN) indicate? The analysis component of the RN exam is the ability to break down the facts and give the rationale for using or applying the facts; for example, What nursing actions are required when a client's lab report has an elevated BUN? According to revised Bloom's *Taxonomy of Educational Objectives* (Anderson & Krathwohl, 2001), analysis is a higher level of cognitive thinking than knowledge, comprehension, and application. Analysis requires the RN to use a higher level of critical thinking to make a judgment regarding the facts or information (see Table 3–1).

In 1989 and 1990, the National League for Nursing (NLN) established roles and responsibilities for practical and associate degree nursing programs.

In 1989 and 1990, the National League for Nursing (NLN) established roles and responsibilities for practical and associate degree nursing programs. The **LPN roles** are detailed as "provider of care," supervised by an RN and "member of the discipline" (Claytor, 1993, p. 228). The **LPN responsibilities** listed under the role *provider of care* are assistance with client assessments and nursing care plans; provision of nursing care; performance of procedures and medication administration;

Table 3–1 NCLEX-PN and NCLEX-RN testing content comparison

Test Plan Element	NCLEX-PN	NCLEX-RN
1. Levels of cognitive ability	Knowledge Comprehension Application Analysis (fewer)	Knowledge (fewer) Comprehension Application Analysis
2. Safe, effective care environment	Coordinate care: Collaborates with other health care team members to facilitate effective client care	Management of care: Providing integrated, cost-effective care to clients by coordinating, supervising, and/or collaborating with members of the multidisciplinary health care team
3. Health promotion and maintenance	Assists the client and significant others in the normal expected stages of growth and development from conception to advanced old age	Provides and directs care that incorporates the knowledge of expected growth and development principles and the prevention and/or early detection of health problems
4. Psychosocial integrity	Promotes the client's ability to cope, adapt, and/or solve situations related to illnesses or stressful events	Provides and directs nursing care that promotes and supports the emotional, mental, and social well-being of the client and significant others
5. Physiological integrity	Provides comfort and assistance in the performance of ADLs	Promotes physical health and well-being by providing care and comfort, reducing client risk potential, and managing the client's health alterations

communication with clients, client families, and health care team members; and documentation. The LPN works under the direction of the RN. The LPN responsibilities listed under the role *member of the discipline* are recognition of personal strengths and weakness in relationship to continued educational needs, potential career mobility, and ethical and legal guidelines. The **RN roles** are "provider of care, manager of care, and member of the profession" (Claytor, 1993, p. 228). The **RN responsibilities** listed under the role *provider of care* are initiation, updating, and completion of nursing assessment and nursing care plans, provision of safe nursing care, initiation and completion of discharge planning, utilization of communication techniques including client teaching plans, and documentation. The RN responsibilities listed under *manager of care* are supervision of client assignments and staff, coordination of client conferences, and maintenance of communication with the health care team. The RN responsibilities listed under *member of profession* are maintenance of personal and professional self-development and self-evaluation; maintenance of ethical and legal standards; and participation in research, organizational change process, and quality control measures.

In 2000, the Council of Associate Degree Nursing Competencies Task Force and the National League for Nursing, with the support of the National Organization of Associate Degree Nursing, wrote *Educational Competencies for Graduates of Associate Degree Nursing Programs* (Coxwell & Gillerman). This document defines the competency expectations of associate degree nurses upon graduation from associate degree nursing programs. The core components break down the main functions of a nurse, and the competencies describe the expected abilities, skills, or expertise of a graduate associate degree nurse. This document delineates the **core components and competencies** of the associate degree RN as "professional behaviors, communication, assessment, clinical decision making, caring interventions, teaching and learning, collaboration, and managing care" (Coxwell & Gillerman, 2000, pp. 7–11).

LPN AND RN ROLES COMPARED WITH THE RN CORE COMPONENTS AND COMPETENCIES

In this chapter, the NLN's detailed LPN and RN roles and responsibilities and RN graduate core components and competencies are used to compare the nursing roles of the LPN and the RN. The NLN-defined LPN and RN responsibilities (Table 3–2) are interwoven in the discussion of the expected graduate core components and competencies. This discussion will assist you in gaining an understanding of the similarities and differences between the LPN and the RN roles, responsibilities, and knowledge base.

Table 3–2 LPN and RN roles and responsibilities

Licensed Practical Nurses	Registered Nurses
Provider of Care	Provider of Care
• Assists in patient assessment.	• Initiates and/or completes nursing assessment, interview, & history of patient.
• Assists with the development, evaluation, & modifications of nursing care plans.	• Initiates & updates written nursing care plans.
• Prioritizes nursing care.	
• Gives direct personal care to patients.	• Implements medical & nursing care plans for patients.
• Performs technical & nontechnical procedures.	• Evaluates & revises nursing care plan through continual assessment.
• Administers medications & monitors IV fluids.	• Provides & participates in comprehensive, safe nursing care to patients.
• Assists patients to prepare for diagnostic tests.	• Initiates nursing discharge planning.
• Establishes & maintains therapeutic relationship with patients, families, & significant others.	• Makes referrals for continued care after discharge.
• Receives information from RN.	• Assesses verbal & nonverbal communication of patients, families, & significant others.
• Keeps RN informed.	
• Communicates as appropriate with other health team members.	• Utilizes communication techniques to assist patient in coping with and resolving problems.
• Documents nursing observations & interventions.	• Explains nursing care to patients & nonprofessional personnel.
	• Implements teaching plans specific to patient's level of development, knowledge, & learning needs.
	• Documents nursing care via the nursing process.

Table 3–2 (continued)

Role Not Delineated for LPNs

- Supervises no one.
- Works under the direction of an RN.

Manager of Care

- Prepares patient care assignments.
- Assists in evaluation of auxiliary personnel performance.
- Assists in orientation of new personnel.
- Supervises employees when in charge of patient care.
- Incorporates cost-effective & environmental safety factors into nursing care plan.
- Plans, directs, and coordinates nursing care of a group of patients.
- Initiates, leads, and/or participates in patient-centered conferences.
- Maintains communication & coordination with health care team members.

Member of the Discipline

- Seeks out learning opportunities and continuing education.
- Practices within the ethical/legal framework of nursing.
- Identifies personal potential & considers career mobility options.
- Identifies personal strengths & weaknesses to improve own performance.

Member of the Profession

- Assumes responsibility for self-development & self-evaluation.
- Practices within the ethical/legal framework of nursing.
- Serves as a role model to members of the nursing team.
- Values nursing as a career.
- Participates in research (e.g., gathers data).
- Works within the organizational framework to facilitate change.
- Assists in quality control measures & procedures.
- Supports peers in delivery of health care.
- Utilizes current literature to provide safe care.

(From "Working Effectively with LPN-RN Orientees," by K. Claytor, 1993, *The Journal of Continuing Education in Nursing*, 12 [5], pp. 227–231.)

At the beginning of this chapter, we discussed the fact that the LPN performs many of the same functions as the RN. From this point on, these functions are viewed as the similarities between the LPN and the RN. The differences between the two roles are the professional changes that you will experience during the next few semesters of your educational experience.

Professional Behaviors

In the *Educational Competencies for Graduates of Associate Degree Nursing Programs* (Coxwell & Gillerman, 2000), the definition of **professional behaviors** states that the nurse "adheres to standards of professional practice, is accountable for her/his own actions and behaviors, and practices nursing within legal, ethical, and regulatory frameworks . . . including a concern for others, as demonstrated by caring, valuing the profession of nursing, and participating in ongoing professional development" (p. 7). According to the 1989 description of LPN roles and responsibilities (National League for Nursing, 1989), the LPN demonstrates professional behaviors by seeking continuing education opportunities.

Professional behavior similarities of the LPN and the RN are that both practice within a legal and ethical framework according to their level of practice. Both value caring by providing nursing care to clients and seeking out continuing education opportunities to keep current in nursing practice and knowledge. The RN evaluates personal learning needs and assumes responsibility for continuing education and personal development.

The RN has opportunities to contribute to the profession by gathering research data, facilitating change in the organizational structure, and analyzing and evaluating quality control measures.

The RN has opportunities to contribute to the profession by gathering research data, facilitating change in the organizational structure, and analyzing and evaluating quality control measures. The RN gathers research data individually or as part of a team by distributing, collecting, and analyzing surveys or conducting interviews. She facilitates changes within an organization by following the change process of analyzing a situation, determining the needed change, recommending desired change to administration, and communicating desired change to colleagues. The RN assists with quality-control measures by participating on a committee that develops facility goals, sets goal criteria for the facility to meet, and then evaluates how the facility meets the established criteria. Some of the criteria the quality-control committee may evaluate are charting, provision of care, and medication administration.

Professional Growth Activities

1. Observe an RN collecting data for a research project.
2. Attend a nurse management meeting to observe ways change is implemented within an organization.
3. Observe an RN conducting quality control within a hospital facility.

Box 3–1 Opportunities for professional growth

Communication

The competencies also define **communication** in nursing as "an interactive process through which there is an exchange of information that may occur verbally, non-verbally, in writing, or through information technology" (Coxwell & Gillerman, 2000, p. 7). "Therapeutic communication is an interactive verbal and non-verbal process between the nurse and client that assists the client to cope with change, develop more satisfying interpersonal relationships, and integrate new knowledge and skills" (p. 7). The LPN has the basic skills to communicate with health care team members and clients. The RN's education and knowledge base give her the ability to assess and analyze verbal and nonverbal communication between clients and family members, clients and health care team members, and among health care team members. The RN also utilizes therapeutic communication techniques to assist clients in coping with problems and to solve problems. Both the LPN and the RN communicate with health care team members, but the RN coordinates communication and activities with clients, family members, and various health care team members.

Assessment

> *The in-depth general education and social science classes equip the RN to assess how each of the dimensions of physical, developmental, emotional, psychosocial, cultural, spiritual, and functional status influences and affects the client.*

The competencies define **assessment** as "the collection, analysis, and synthesis of relevant data for the purpose of appraising the client's health status. Comprehensive assessment provides a holistic view of the client which includes dimensions of physical, developmental, emotional, psychosocial, cultural, spiritual, and functional status" (Coxwell & Gillerman, 2000, p. 8). The LPN gathers basic data on each of the previously mentioned assessment dimensions and contributes information for the nursing process (Figure 3–1). The RN does an in-depth assessment, analyzes and synthesizes the information, and utilizes the nursing process steps of goal setting, planning, and interventions to address the client needs. (See appendix B for a more in-depth assessment.) In-depth general education and social science classes equip the RN to assess how each of the dimensions of physical, developmental, emotional, psychosocial, cultural, spiritual, and functional status influences and affects the client.

Clinical Decision Making

The competencies state that **clinical decision making** "encompasses the performance of accurate assessments, the use of multiple methods to access information, and the analysis and integration of knowledge and information to formulate clinical judgments" (Coxwell & Gillerman, 2000, p. 8). The LPN assists in client assessments and works under the direction of the RN. The RN performs more comprehensive, in-depth assessments obtained from multiple sources and then applies critical thinking to determine the best client care approach.

> *The RN performs more comprehensive, in-depth assessments obtained from multiple sources and then applies critical thinking to determine the best client care approach.*

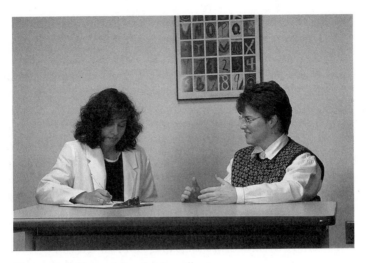

Figure 3–1 Nurse interviewing client.

Caring Interventions

The competencies define **caring interventions** as "those nursing behaviors and actions that assist clients in meeting their needs . . . based on a knowledge and understanding of the natural sciences, behavioral sciences, nursing theory, nursing research, and past nursing experiences. . . . Caring behaviors are nurturing, protective, compassionate, and person-centered" (Coxwell & Gillerman, 2000, p. 9). Both LPNs and RNs provide excellent caring interventions to clients. The RN has more in-depth knowledge of natural sciences, behavioral sciences, nursing theory, and nursing research that enables her to have a more holistic view of the client.

Teaching and Learning

An RN assesses the needs of the client and then develops an individualized client teaching plan.

The competencies state that **teaching** "encompasses the provision of health education to promote and facilitate informed decision making, achieve positive outcomes, and support self-care activities. Integral components of the teaching process include the transmission of information, evaluation of the response to teaching, and modification of teaching based on identified responses" (Coxwell & Gillerman, 2000, pp. 9–10). The competencies also state that **learning** "involves the assimilation of information to expand knowledge and change behavior" (Coxwell & Gillerman, 2000, p. 10). An RN would fulfill these responsibilities by assessing the needs of the client and then developing an individualized client teaching plan (Figure 3–2).

Learning outcomes are set for the client and then the RN evaluates the client's progress toward those learning outcomes. The RN modifies the teaching plan according to the client's progress in expanded knowledge and observed changed behaviors. Teaching responsibilities of the LPN are not mentioned in the 1989 competencies. However, the LPN assists with some client teaching under the direction of the RN. The depth of teaching increases as the nurse obtains more education.

Collaboration

The competencies define **collaboration** as "the shared planning, decision making, problem solving, goal setting, and assumption of responsibilities by those who work together cooperatively, with open professional communication" (Coxwell & Gillerman, 2000, p. 10). The LPN is part of the collaborating team, but the RN initiates and directs the planning, decision making, problem solving, and goal setting of the collaborative process. The LPN assists with the planning, decision making, problem solving, and goal setting.

Managing Care

The RN completes client care assignments; orients, supervises, and evaluates staff performance; is in charge of client care; coordinates care for a group of clients; includes safety and cost-effective factors in the clients' care plans; and leads individualized client conferences.

The competencies define **managing care** as "the efficient, effective use of human, physical, financial, and technological resources to meet client needs and support organizational outcomes" (Coxwell & Gillerman, 2000, p. 10). According to the NLN's LPN roles and responsibilities, the LPN's managing care consists of assisting with client assessments;

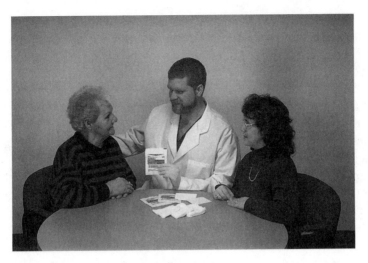

Figure 3–2 Nurse teaching client.

assisting with the development, evaluation, and modification of nursing care plans; prioritizing nursing care; and giving direct client care. The LPN works under the direction of an RN and supervises certified nursing assistants. The RN initiates and completes the nursing assessment including the client interview and history; initiates, evaluates, and revises written nursing care plans; and initiates discharge planning. The RN includes community resources in the discharge planning according to the assessed physical, psychosocial, and financial needs of the client. The RN completes client care assignments; orients, supervises, and evaluates staff performance; is in charge of client care; coordinates care for a group of clients; includes safety and cost-effective factors in the clients' care plans; and leads individualized client conferences.

$\mathcal{S}$UMMARY

The rationale for performing a procedure in a certain way is based on knowledge and critical thinking skills gained through the educational experience of the RN.

In transitioning from LPN to RN, it may be necessary for the LPN to rethink the concept that the LPN does everything the RN does. The LPN does perform some of the same procedures as the RN; the difference between the LPN and the RN is the rationale for performing a procedure in a certain way. The rationale is based on knowledge and critical thinking skills gained through the educational experience of the RN. In other words, the reason a procedure varies slightly between one client and another is determined by nursing judgment and critical thinking based on in-depth scientific principles and psychological and social issues involving the client. These skills are gained from the general education and social science classes required in the associate degree program. There are many similarities in the procedures that LPNs and RNs perform; the differences are rooted in the knowledge base and critical thinking skills that include analysis, modification, assimilation, synthesis, problem solving, and evaluation.

You now have an opportunity to transition into the RN role with higher levels of performance and reasoning.

You have demonstrated your competence as an LPN, or you would not be enrolled in an associate degree nursing program. Your educational experience in the next few semesters will assist you in developing the needed critical thinking skills. Maria Gomez, as a new LPN to RN graduate, said her toughest transition to RN "was accepting the autonomy and authority of an RN" (personal communication, May 13, 2003).

"The greatest impediment to future success in a new role is inability to relinquish your old one" (Porter-O'Grady, 1999, p. 8). You now have an opportunity to transition into the RN role with higher levels of performance and reasoning.

CRITICAL THINKING ACTIVITY

1. Observe an RN performing each of the following role components. Record what you observe as the main differences in the LPN role and the RN role.

   • Professional behaviors:

   _____

   _____

   _____

   _____

- Communication:

_____

_____

_____

_____

- Assessment:

_____

_____

_____

_____

- Clinical decision making:

_____

_____

_____

_____

- Caring interventions:

_____

_____

_____

_____

- Teaching and learning:

_____

_____

_____

_____

- Collaboration:

_____

_____

_____

_____

- Managing care:

_____

_____

_____

_____

ℭHAPTER REFLECTIONS

1. What nursing practices do you expect to change as you become an RN? You may want to consider concepts such as professional behaviors, communication, assessment, decision making, client teaching and client learning, collaboration, and managing care.

2. How do you think your education and role as an RN will assist you in making decisions related to client care?

3. Describe the RN you most admire. What qualities does she or he possess that you want to make part of your own nursing practice? How do these qualities differ from your current nursing behavior?

REFERENCES

Anderson, L., & Krathwohl, D. (2001). *A taxonomy for learning, teaching and assessing: A revision of Bloom's taxonomy of educational objectives.* New York: Longman.

Chornick, N., Yocom, C., & Jacobson, J. (1993). *1993 job analysis study of newly licensed entry-level registered nurses.* Chicago: National Council of State Boards of Nursing.

Claytor, K. (1993). Working effectively with LPN-RN orientees. *The Journal of Continuing Education in Nursing, 12*(5), 227–231.

Coxwell, G., and Gillerman, H. (Eds.). (2000). *Educational competencies for graduates of associate degree nursing programs.* Sudbury, MA: Jones and Bartlett Publishers.

Kane, M., & Colton, D. (1988). *Job analysis of newly licensed practical/vocational nurses: 1986–87.* Chicago: National Council of State Boards of Nursing.

National Council of State Boards of Nursing. (1989). *Test plan for the national council licensure examination for practical nurses (NCLEX-PN).* Chicago: Author.

National Council of State Boards of Nursing. (1994). *Test plan for the national council licensure examination for registered nurses (NCLEX-RN).* Chicago: Author.

National Council of State Boards of Nursing. (2000). *NCSBN testplans for NCLEX-RN® and NCLEX-PN®.* Chicago: Author.

National League for Nursing: Council of Practical Nursing Programs. (1989). *Entry-level competencies of graduates of educational programs in practical nursing.* New York: Author.

National League for Nursing. (1990). *Educational outcomes of associate degree nursing programs: Roles and competencies.* New York: Author.

Porter-O'Grady, T. (1999). Technology demands quick-change nursing roles. *Nursing Management, 30*(5), 7–8.

SUGGESTED RESOURCES

Meehan, M. (1999). Nursing roles: Advice, counseling, or therapy? *Paediatric Nursing, 11*(6), 30–36.

Pope, B. (2002). The synergy match-up. *Nursing Management, 33*(5), 38–41.

Rick, C. (2003). Differentiated practice: Get beyond the fear factor. *Nursing Management, 34*(1), 11–12.

Warden-Saunders, J. (1999). Nursing's role. *Nursing Homes, 48*(12), 106–108.

$\mathscr{P}$ART II
The Nurse as Caregiver

▼ ▼ ▼ ▼ ▼ ▼ ▼

Chapter 4
Provider of Care

▼ ▼ ▼ ▼ ▼ ▼ ▼

LEARNING OBJECTIVES

By the end of this chapter, you should be able to:

1. Define caring.
2. Explain the relationship of caring to nursing practice.
3. List some goals of nursing practice.

KEY TERM

Caring

SCENARIO

Kerry, a 22-year-old male, is one day post-op from an ileostomy for the treatment of Crohn's disease. He is feeling anxious and has many questions about care of the ileostomy and the lifestyle changes that he will have to make. He has total parenteral nutrition (TPN) infusing through his central line, a patient-controlled analgesia (PCA) pump, a Jackson-Pratt (JP) drain, and a new ileostomy and its appliance. The alarm has just gone off on the intravenous (IV) pump, and Kerry is experiencing increased pain at the stoma site.

Jamie, a cheerful young nurse, enters Kerry's room with a smile. While offering support and encouragement, she attempts to determine the problem with the IV. She finds the alarm silence button but is unable to restart the IV, affecting the administration of both the TPN and pain control. When Kerry groans with pain, the nurse begins to assess him; she finds a discoloration in the stoma and recognizes that the physician needs to be notified. Unsure of what else to do to correct the problem, Jamie tells Kerry she will need to get assistance. She returns shortly with her mentor nurse, Jack. Jack does not smile or speak to Kerry but quickly attends to the technical equipment. Then he checks the stoma, again without speaking or making any connection with the client. He tends to all of Kerry's needs in a timely manner. Jack is obviously very technically competent and knowledgeable about the post-op care of a new ostomy client.

*T*HINK ABOUT IT

1. Compare and contrast the care provided by the two nurses, Jamie and Jack, in the preceding scenario.
2. Which nurse would you prefer to have care for you? Why?
3. Define *caring* as it relates to nursing.

*I*NTRODUCTION

Is the concept of caring included in your list of words that describe a good nurse? With advances in technology, do you think the personal touch has been diminishing in nursing practice? In this chapter we will discuss the relationship of caring and nursing practice, and we will list goals of nursing practice as they relate to caring.

CRITICAL THINKING ACTIVITY

Complete the caring survey in Figure 4–1 to examine your thoughts on caring and nursing.

1. What new concepts of caring as a nurse did you discover as you completed the caring survey?

_____

_____

_____

CARING EFFICACY SCALE*

INSTRUCTIONS: When you are completing these items, think of your recent work with patients/clients in clinical settings. Circle the number that best expresses your opinion.

Rating Scale:

-3 Strongly disagree	+1 Slightly agree
-2 Moderately disagree	+2 Moderately agree
-1 Slightly dissagree	+3 Strongly agree

	Strongly disagree			Strongly agree		
1. I do not feel confident in my ability to express a sense of caring to my clients/patients.	- 3	- 2	- 1	+ 1	+2	+3
2. If I am not relating well to a client/patient, I try to analyze what I can do to reach him/her.	- 3	- 2	- 1	+ 1	+2	+3
3. I feel comfortable in touching my clients/patients in the course of caregiving.	- 3	- 2	- 1	+ 1	+2	+3
4. I convey a sense of personal strength to my clients/patients.	- 3	- 2	- 1	+ 1	+2	+3
5. Clients/patients can tell me most anything and I won't be shocked.	- 3	- 2	- 1	+ 1	+2	+3
6. I have an ability to introduce a sense of normalcy in stressful conditions.	- 3	- 2	- 1	+ 1	+2	+3
7. It is easy for me to consider the multifacets of a client's/patient's care, at the same time as I am listening to them.	- 3	- 2	- 1	+ 1	+2	+3
8. I have difficulty in suspending my personal beliefs and biases in order to hear and accept a client/patient as a person.	- 3	- 2	- 1	+ 1	+2	+3
9. I can walk into a room with a presence of serenity and energy that makes clients/patients feel better.	- 3	- 2	- 1	+ 1	+2	+3
10. I am able to tune into a particular client/patient and forget my personal concerns.	- 3	- 2	- 1	+ 1	+2	+3
11. I can usually create some way to relate to most any client/patient.	- 3	- 2	- 1	+ 1	+2	+3
12. I lack confidence in my ability to talk to clients/patients from backgrounds different from my own.	- 3	- 2	- 1	+ 1	+2	+3

Figure 4–1 Caring efficacy scale. (continues)

	Strongly disagree			Strongly agree		
13. I feel if I talk to clients/patients on an individual, personal basis, things might get out of control.	-3	-2	-1	+1	+2	+3
14. I use what I learn in conversations with clients/patients to provide more individualized care.	-3	-2	-1	+1	+2	+3
15. I don't feel strong enough to listen to the fears and concerns of my clients/patients.	-3	-2	-1	+1	+2	+3
16. Even when I'm feeling self-confident about most things, I still seem to be unable to relate to clients/patients.	-3	-2	-1	+1	+2	+3
17. I seem to have trouble relating to clients/patients.	-3	-2	-1	+1	+2	+3
18. I can usually establish a close relationship with my clients/patients.	-3	-2	-1	+1	+2	+3
19. I can usually get patients/clients to like me.	-3	-2	-1	+1	+2	+3
20. I often find it hard to get my point of view across to patients/clients when I need to.	-3	-2	-1	+1	+2	+3
21. When trying to resolve a conflict with a client/patient, I usually make it worse.	-3	-2	-1	+1	+2	+3
22. If I think a client/patient is uneasy or may need some help, I approach that person.	-3	-2	-1	+1	+2	+3
23. If I find it hard to relate to a client/patient, I'll stop trying to work with that person.	-3	-2	-1	+1	+2	+3
24. I often find it hard to relate to clients/patients from a different culture than mine.	-3	-2	-1	+1	+2	+3
25. I have helped many clients/patients through my ability to develop close, meaningful relationships.	-3	-2	-1	+1	+2	+3
26. I often find it difficult to express empathy with clients/patients.	-3	-2	-1	+1	+2	+3
27. I often become overwhelmed by the nature of the problems clients/patients are experiencing.	-3	-2	-1	+1	+2	+3
28. When a client/patient is having difficulty communicating with me, I am able to adjust to his/her level.	-3	-2	-1	+1	+2	+3

Figure 4–1 (continues)

	Strongly disagree			Strongly agree		
29. Even when I really try, I can't get through to difficult clients/patients.	- 3	- 2	- 1	+ 1	+2	+3
30. I don't use creative or unusual ways to express caring to my clients/patients.	- 3	- 2	- 1	+ 1	+2	+3

(Permission of Carolie J. Coates, Ph.D., Research Consultant, 1441 Snowmass Court, Boulder, Co. 80305.) © The Caring Efficacy Scale (CES) is copyrighted. This is the 30-item self-report form. Please contact Carolie J. Coates, Ph.D., Research and Measurement Consultant, 1441 Snowmass Court, Boulder, Colorado, 80305, U.S.A., to formally request to use the Caring Efficacy Scale 9CES). (An administrator/supervisor version [30-items] is also available, as well as short forms [12-items] of the self-report and administrator/supervisor version.) Telephone and Fax +(303) 499-5756 E-mail: coatescj@home.com (1/9/2001).

Figure 4–1 (continued)

ARING

> *Caring is a deep-seated involvement in the lives of others; a commitment to provide quality care, to assist the client to a quality state of health, or a presence as the client dies with dignity.*

Since the days of Florence Nightingale, there has been a direct link between nursing and service to others (Kearney, 2001). When nursing students are asked why they want to become a nurse, they frequently respond, "To help others." This response partially defines caring because caring cannot occur if others are not involved. Caring requires a recipient.

Caring is a deep-seated involvement in the lives of others; a commitment to provide quality care, to assist the client to a quality state of health, or a presence as the client dies with dignity. Caring is a complex, observable fact and experience.

Caring as the Core of Nursing

Several theorists have developed conceptual models based on caring. They include Dorthea Orem's Self-Care Deficit Model (1995), Jean

Watson's Human Science and Human Care Model (1999), and Madeleine Leininger's Culture Care Diversity and Universality (2001). Orem believes that all individuals desire to care for and meet their personal care needs and that each person has varied abilities to participate in meeting his personal self-care needs. The nurse attempts to meet the client's self-care needs in an effort to reduce the client's self-care deficits. Watson believes that caring is a moral ideal and that nursing is a caring art and science. The client is the center of human caring. Leininger believes that nursing is a learned art focused on caring in accord with an individual's culture. To these theorists, caring definitely is a component of nursing.

Nursing research indicates that nurses and clients identify different concepts when defining *caring* in the provision of care. To Bertero (1999) caring includes "all aspects of delivering nursing care to patients" (p. 414). Caring is the heart and unifying core of nursing. Theorist Leininger proposes that caring is the trademark of nursing practice: "Care is the essence and the central unifying and dominant domain to characterize nursing. Care has also been postulated to be an essential human need for the full development, health maintenance, and survival of human beings in all world cultures" (1988, p. 3). These statements imply that caring is the very essence of nursing care and at the core of nursing practice.

Caring also is a basic human need that must be fulfilled if an individual is to obtain his full potential. Nurses can meet a client's needs when providing nursing care. "Caring is a commitment by the nurse to become involved, and its character is relational. Nurses enter this relationship with their whole being" (Bertero, 1999, p. 415).

"The nurse's role is 'being with' rather than 'doing to' a patient" (Bertero, 1999, p. 415). Clients expect competence in performing procedures. Nurses provide competent care when they adeptly perform procedures and are "with" the client relationally during the procedure. The nurse can also be with or "connected to" the client when the client needs to talk or share intimate personal feelings. "Caring means connecting with clients by listening to their thoughts and fears, and communicating concern" (p. 415). Caring is more than a physical presence, it is a relational concern for the other's well-being.

Caring Defined by Caring Experiences

A research project analyzed the narrative writing of 68 nursing students as they described caring experiences (Schaefer, 2002). From the study, five themes were identified:

1. Nurses need to care for themselves to care for others.
2. Emotional attachment has dangers.
3. Caring involves a moral responsibility.
4. Reflections on care teach about caring.
5. Reflection engages one in defining caring. (p. 3)

In the first theme, the students identified their need to receive care in order to prepare them to care for others. As the students experienced caring in personal situations, they learned the value of receiving care and also acquired a desire to meet others' needs by caring for them. The caring process is a continuous, ongoing process. An individual receives care, then gives care to another, who learns about care and then gives care to another. Our life experiences in which we receive care prepare us for future caring opportunities. In this way, nurses who receive care learn and are equipped to give care.

The second theme, that emotional attachment has dangers, is described (Schaefer, 2002) in a situation in which a client started to cry, causing an emotional response from the student that led to the student's bursting into tears. The student was then incapable of meeting the physical or emotional needs of his client (p. 289). Nurses walk a tightrope between caring and tempering their emotions to provide competent care. Emotional attachment spurs caring, but emotional attachment can be painful, difficult, and a hindrance to adequate care. Nurses learn to balance these emotions with experience and growth.

The third theme emphasizes that caring is a moral responsibility. As nurses become aware of the needs of others, they have to make a choice. Do they meet the need, or do they ignore the need? In that decision lies the moral choice or responsibility. Hopefully, in becoming aware of another's need, the nurse comprehends and has an emotional response to the client's situation and is motivated to respond with conscious, caring, appropriate actions to address the client's situation.

The choice to respond with caring actions is self-giving and will cost the nurse something—time, energy, or possibly convenience—but responding positively to a moral choice is self-satisfying and personally responsible.

The fourth theme supports the idea that as we reflect on caring experiences, we learn about caring. As the students pondered their client caring experiences, one student realized that she had cared for a client for several days but had not really gotten to know her particular likes and dislikes. The author recently observed a similar situation, in which a nurse offered a client a nutrition tray with the regular tea provided by the facility, but another nurse who had taken the time to get to know the client was aware that the client preferred a special tea she had stored in her bedside drawer. One student stated that her caring experience could be labeled "caring, patient advocacy, or simply my job" (Schaefer, 2002, p. 290) How would the environment of a facility change if all nurses provided genuine care because caring was "simply my job?"

CRITICAL THINKING ACTIVITY

1. Describe a time when you showed caring in your role as a nurse. Describe the events leading to the interaction, your interaction with the client, and the result of the interaction (Schaefer, 2002).

   _____

   _____

   _____

   _____

   _____

2. After writing about your caring experience, share what you learned about caring with your classmates.

Caring is seen not as a duty but as an actual giving of self to establish a relationship with another.

Acts of Caring

Bertero (1999) conducted a qualitative research study of nurses' sharing their experiences in situations when caring was given to a client and was not given to a client. The theme that emerged from the nurses' sharing their caring experiences was the development and maintenance of a "helping-trusting interpersonal relationship" (p. 416). This relationship was maintained in five ways, or subthemes:

1. Creation of an interaction with the client and next of kin.
2. Actions to satisfy the needs of the client and next of kin.
3. Feelings of frustration in the caring role.
4. Influence of time constraints.
5. Development of self and gaining insight (Bertero, 1999).

The first subtheme, creating an interaction with the client and next of kin, included verbal and nonverbal communication and touch. The interactions could include eye contact that says "I know" or "I care," or compassionately placing a hand on the client's forearm to say "I care." "Creating interaction is not just a task: It is making contact, relating and being present with the patients and their next of kin" (Bertero, 1999, p. 417). Caring is seen not as a duty but as an actual giving of self to establish a relationship with another. When have you given of yourself to establish a professional relationship with a client? This emotional interaction can be extremely rewarding.

The second subtheme, acting to satisfy the needs of the client and next of kin, includes recognizing and anticipating the client's physical, emotional, social, and spiritual needs. These are actions of competence, service, presence, and respect for the client and next of kin.

Frustrating feelings in the caring role, the third subtheme, were experienced when unclear, unrealistic, or false information was given to the client and next of kin. The nurses also experienced frustration when they could do nothing to save the client's life. It was then that the client was assisted with a comforting, peaceful, and dignified death.

In the fourth subtheme, nurses felt that time constraints influenced their ability to care for a client. They also felt limited by the brevity of some lives and attempted to improve quality in the time frame available.

Quality could take the form of fluffing a pillow for comfort, attentively listening to a client's sharing past experiences with children, or assisting a client in forgiving a past hurt.

The fifth subtheme was nurses' experiencing self-development and gaining insight. "The nurses stated that when they viewed themselves as competent in caring and obtaining satisfaction from the patient, they developed their sense of self and improved their self-esteem" (Bertero, 1999, p. 419). The nurses felt that they gained insight from client interactions and viewing clients' life experiences. Caring is truly a two-way, relational experience. It is a complex experience involving personal interaction and competence in skilled techniques.

CRITICAL THINKING ACTIVITIES

1. Share a personal experience when you:

   • Interacted with a client and his or her next of kin.

   _____
   _____
   _____

   • Acted to satisfy the needs of a client and his or her next of kin.

   _____
   _____
   _____

   • Felt frustrated in the caring role.

   _____
   _____
   _____

   • Felt the influence of time constraints when caring for a client.

   _____
   _____
   _____
   _____

   • Developed your sense of self and gained personal insight.

   _____
   _____
   _____

2. What were the dynamics that made the interaction a positive experience?

_____

_____

_____

3. How could the experience have been improved?

_____

_____

_____

GOALS OF NURSING PRACTICE

Nursing, to a professional, is a career plan, a central part of his or her core being; and caring is the behavioral outcome.

To some nurses, nursing provides financial reward. To others, nursing provides self-satisfaction or self-fulfillment. To still others, nursing defines who they are. Nursing, to a professional, is a career plan, a central part of his core being; and caring is the behavioral outcome.

The concepts of essential relationships and self-reward may comprise care of others and care of self. "Components of this service ideal include a profound sense of purpose, a true sense of capability, and a deep concern for others demonstrated as caring" (Hood & Leddy, 2003, p. 32). Service to others provides a meaningful life purpose. Service gives the individual feelings of competence in the ability to perform a task. Service is the link between concern for others and action in response to concern.

SUMMARY

The goals of nursing practice combine knowledge, self-care, and competent technical skills. Caring is providing competent physical, emotional, and spiritual care; interacting verbally and nonverbally with clients and their families; satisfying the needs of clients and their families; and experiencing self-development and gaining personal insight. Nursing is "caring from the heart . . . and the head." Nurses should "exercise their intellectual skills to provide the best care possible. . . . Nurses who constantly think, as well as feel for their patients, are the best nurses." The best nurses are those "who are smart critical thinkers, who are constantly questioning what is best for the patient, what is best for the organization, is there a better way?" (Curran, 1999, p. 73). The union of caring and competence are the goals of nursing practice. Nursing is defined as an art and a science. Nursing is the "science of caring" (Huch, 2003, p. 82).

CRITICAL THINKING ACTIVITY

After reading this chapter, write your own definitions of the terms *nursing practice, caring,* and *competence.*

1. Nursing practice: _____
   _____
   _____

2. Caring: _____
   _____
   _____

3. Competence: _____
   _____
   _____

*C*HAPTER REFLECTIONS

1. We have said that the goals of nursing practice are a combination of knowledge, caring, and competent technical skills. List your personal goals of nursing practice.

2. What role does caring have in your nursing practice?

REFERENCES

Bertero, C. (1999). Caring for and about cancer patients: Identifying the meaning of the phenomenon "caring" through narratives. *Cancer Nursing, 22*(6), 414–420.

Coates, C. (2002). Caring Efficacy Scale. In J. Watson, *Assessing and measuring caring in nursing and health science* (pp. 171–173). New York: Springer Publishing Company.

Curran, C. (1999). Caring for the heart . . . and the head. *Nursing Economics, 17*(2), 73.

Hood, L., and Leddy, S. (2003). *Leddy and Pepper's conceptual bases of professional nursing* (5th ed.). Philadelphia: Lippincott.

Huch, M. (2003). The many facets of caring. *Nursing Science Quarterly, 16*(1), 82–83.

Kearney, R. (2001). *Advancing your career: Concepts of professional nursing.* Philadelphia: F.A. Davis Company.

Leininger, M. (1988). *Care: The essence of nursing and health.* Detroit, MI: Wayne State University Press.

Leininger, M. (1995). *Transcultural nursing* (2nd ed.). New York: McGraw-Hill.

Leininger, M. (2001). *Culture care diversity and universality: A theory of nursing.* Boston: Jones and Bartlett.

Orem, D. (1995). *Nursing: Concepts of practice* (5th ed.). St. Louis: Mosby.

Schaefer, K. (2002). Reflections on caring narratives: Enhancing patterns of knowing. *Nursing Education Perspectives, 23,* 286–293.

Watson, J. (1999). *Nursing: Human science and human care* (3rd ed.). Norwalk, CT: Appleton-Century-Crofts.

SUGGESTED RESOURCES

Huffman, D., Lewis, S., & Nelson, M. (2002). Advancing technology, caring, and nursing. *Nursing Science Quarterly, 15*(4), 434–437.

Mustard, L. (2002). Caring and competency. *JONA's Healthcare Law, Ethics, and Regulation, 4,* 36–43.

*C*hapter 5
Clinical Decision Making
and the Nursing Process

▼ ▼ ▼ ▼ ▼ ▼ ▼

*L*EARNING OBJECTIVES

By the end of this chapter, you should be able to:

1. Define the stages of clinical judgment.
2. Explain the steps in problem solving.
3. Explain the steps in decision making.
4. Explain the steps in the nursing process.
5. Develop a care plan using the steps in the nursing process.

*K*EY TERMS

Assessment
Clinical judgment
Decision making
Decision tree
Evaluating
Gantt chart
Implementing
Nursing diagnosis
Nursing interventions
Nursing process
PERT chart
Planning nursing care
Problem solving

*S*CENARIO

Tameka has been a nurse on a medical surgical unit for three months. Her client experienced left arm pain, nausea, shortness of breath, and diaphoresis three days postoperatively. She medicated the client for pain, but the pain was not relieved by the medication. She sought advice from a more experienced nurse on the unit who had her call the doctor because she was concerned that the client was experiencing symptoms of a heart attack. Tameka feels bad that she did not recognize these symptoms. She feels like an incompetent nurse and that maybe she should just quit.

*T*HINK ABOUT IT

1. Should new nurses be expected to determine what is happening with a patient from observed signs and symptoms in all cases?
2. Does seeking advice from a co-worker make you an incompetent nurse?
3. Did Tameka respond in an appropriate manner?

*I*NTRODUCTION

It is critical for nurses to make quick, accurate, and effective decisions. In this chapter we will discuss the steps in clinical judgment, problem solving, and decision making. The nursing process is the nursing discipline's method of assisting nurses in making decisions, so the steps of the nursing process are explained in detail with an opportunity for the student to complete a nursing care plan.

*C*LINICAL JUDGMENT

Benner et al. (1996) suggest that clinical judgment progresses from a novice stage to an expert stage.

Benner, Tanner, and Chesla (1996) propose that "the clinical judgment of experienced nurses resembles much more . . . engaged practical reasoning . . . than the disengaged, scientific, or theoretical reasoning . . . represented in the nursing process" (p. 1). They suggest that

clinical judgment progresses from a novice stage to an expert stage. Their theory, known as the five-stage novice-to-expert practice model, is based on inductive studies of clinical practice settings. Benner et al.'s model proposes that an experienced nurse gains understanding of and responds to a person's illness by knowing the client and by having gained proficient clinical knowledge through the experience of caring for many persons in similar situations, rather than by labeling a client with a nursing diagnosis. The experiential clinical knowledge makes the nurse more aware of possible issues and concerns that could occur in other similar clinical situations. Hood and Leddy (2003) state, "this [Benner et al.'s] model is individualized rather than rule based, and emphasizes the integration of nonconscious, nonanalytical aspects of judgment, experience, and reflection on rational critical thinking" (p. 253). Benner et al.'s model encourages the nurse to view the client as an individual with individual issues and concerns instead of applying a set of rules to each client's situation.

It is important to remember that each client's response to a situation will vary and requires a different approach in the care provided. For example, two clients enter the health care setting with pneumonia. The basic treatment for each client is the same, but each client has varying issues and concerns that require different clinical approaches. For instance, one may have good-quality insurance and not be worried about the medical bills, and the other may have postponed seeing a physician because of financial concerns. The clients may vary in age, and the elder require more intensive therapy. Both clients have pneumonia, but one client's is uncomplicated, and the other, elderly client has a history of asthma, and emphysema. The nurse's clinical approach obviously will differ with each of these clients.

As the nurse progresses through the novice to expert stages, she begins to rely on her internal instincts along with her clinical judgment and experience in the critical thinking process. If the nurse is attuned to her instincts, she may sense the client's financial concerns and collaborate with the facilities' social services department. Or she may recall, from previous experience with other seriously ill clients, that advanced directives should be addressed with an elderly client with pneumonia, asthma, and emphysema. Each of these clients may have the same basic nursing diagnoses, but the nurse varies the clinical interventions to meet the client's individual needs.

CRITICAL THINKING ACTIVITY

1. Review the clinical judgment section and identify the key components related to clinical judgment that you think are important. Note the passages quoted from Benner et al. and Hood and Leddy. How will these components change your clinical judgment?

_____

_____

_____

Stages of Clinical Judgment

The five stages of Benner et al.'s model of clinical judgment (1996) are novice, advanced beginner, competent, proficient, and expert.

Novice Stage

The novice focuses on the task and memorizes the rules to complete the task successfully.

The novice stage occurs during the education process (Benner et al., 1996). The novice is presented with tasks that are to be completed by a standard set of rules or guidelines. The novice focuses on the task and memorizes the rules to complete the task successfully. The context in which the task occurs is not totally seen by the novice at this point. For example, when learning to transfer a stroke client with left-side involvement from the bed to a wheelchair, the novice learns as many rules as possible, such as placing the wheelchair on the client's uninvolved side (in this case, the right side) and locking the wheelchair wheels before transferring the client.

Advanced Beginner Stage

The advanced beginner sees the clinical experience as a list of tasks to complete in an organized, prioritized manner.

During the advanced beginner stage (Benner et al., 1996), the nurse begins to recognize the surroundings in which tasks are completed. The advanced beginner nurse has gained experience and has learned more rules for handling the tasks. She begins to recognize difficult situations when performing tasks and sees the tasks as more difficult. Clinically, the advanced beginner is anxious, perhaps somewhat overwhelmed, and she sees the clinical experience as a list of tasks to complete in an organized, prioritized manner. The advanced beginner has a fragmented view of the situation and is dependent on the knowledge and skills of others. She does not see herself as a participant in the overall situation. She views her clinical practice as a set of external standards or orders that test her personal abilities. She is uncertain of her ability to contribute to the overall clinical situation. For example, consider a new nurse who is caring for a renal dialysis client. She knows the classification, action, side effects, and nursing considerations of the client's medications, but she is uncertain if these medications should be given prior to, during, or following dialysis. She needs to consult with a more experienced RN for guidance in medication administration.

Competent Stage

In the competent stage, the nurse has gained organizational and technical skill and approaches client care with a plan that assists in making decisions about the client's condition.

In the competent stage, the nurse has gained organizational and technical skill and approaches client care with a plan that assists in making decisions about the client's condition. She feels confident and competent in her nursing care. She knows she can no longer function totally by rules and memorized steps but needs to see the client's individual needs and assess her overall physical condition. She then analyzes all of the obtained data and makes a decision or seeks another health care provider's input. In the advanced beginner stage, we used the example of a nurse caring for a renal dialysis client who knew something about the client's medication but was not knowledgeable about administering it. In the competent stage, the nurse knows what medications to give and when the medications should be given in relationship to dialysis. She completes thorough assessments of the client and recognizes the rationale behind complications. For example, if a client returned to the floor with slight hypotension, the competent nurse would know why dialysis clients may have hypotension after dialysis but might have difficulty determining when or if to give the hypertensive medication. She might have to refer to a more experienced colleague for advice on when or if to give the hypertensive medication.

Proficient Stage

> *The proficient nurse intuitively determines the importance of various factors in situations.*

The proficient nurse intuitively determines the importance of various factors in situations. The nurse differentiates patterns and anticipates needed actions in client situations. Emotional and reasoned decisions of nursing options in these situations are easier and less stressful, but decisions are still based on rules. The nurse interacts with the clients and families with acquired, wide-ranging skills. An example is a nurse receiving a report from surgery that a client who had a thyroidectomy is returning to the floor. The nurse checks the computer for clinical skills of a post-op thyroidectomy client and then orders a tracheostomy tray to the floor to be available in case of an emergency. The nurse prepares the family prior to bringing the tracheostomy tray into the room so that the family will not become overly concerned.

Expert Stage

> *The expert nurse uses discernment and critical thinking based on experienced intuition, observations, and non-emotional, practical reasoning.*

The expert nurse uses discernment and critical thinking based on experienced intuition, observations, and non-emotional, practical reasoning. She relies on theory or asks other expert nurses for advice. She sees the big picture and anticipates and responds to potential complications. In the proficient stage example, the nurse used the computer to gather data on caring for a post-op thyroidectomy client. In the expert stage, the nurse in the same situation, without mentally reviewing steps of care, would immediately order the tracheostomy tray to the floor and prepare the family for the client's return to the room.

CRITICAL THINKING ACTIVITY

1. Review the examples related to each stage of clinical judgment. Do you think the examples in each stage appropriately represent the actions of a nurse in that stage?

_____

_____

_____

2. Determine your placement in the five-stage novice-to-expert practice model. Support your decision by relating appropriate statements from this text to two personal clinical examples.

_____

_____

_____

$\mathcal{P}$ROBLEM SOLVING

Problem solving is thoroughly analyzing a problem or situation and looking at multiple options in determining the best solution.

We are confronted daily with problems and situations in which we have to seek the best solution. **Problem solving** is thoroughly analyzing a problem or situation and looking at multiple options in determining the best solution to the problem. Problem solving involves using critical thinking skills that lead to the most effective solution. According to Tomey (2000), the steps in problem solving (revised) are: identify the problem, generate possible solutions and examine suggested solutions, choose the best solution, implement the chosen solution, and evaluate the effectiveness of the solution and whether the problem has been resolved. These steps can be followed in solving personal, professional, or client problems.

Identify the Problem

Sometimes problems that surface are not the root of the problem, but symptoms of the root. We need to gather all available information by asking questions of and seeking information from several sources. We must be open to all sides of the issue, regardless of the personalities or personal issues involved. The nurse needs to examine her personal

feelings and thoughts about the issue to be sure that they do not interfere with finding the best solution. These actions allow the nurse to get
to the root of the problem. If the root is not defined and addressed, the
problem may resurface at a later time.

Generate Possible Solutions and Examine Suggested Solutions

Once you have identified the problem, generate as many solutions as
possible. It is important to brainstorm ideas regardless of how irrational
or crazy they may appear at first. Some of the best solutions are created
when we feel free to think outside the box. Explore the future ramifications of all suggested solutions. What will be the potential results of
each one? Which solutions are viable, and which ones are not?

Choose the Best Solution

Some decisions are hard to make because the consequences will not be
pleasant for all persons involved. The best solution is chosen only after
you have reviewed all data and all possible solutions. A common scenario for this decision-making process is a family with a terminally ill
member. The spouse is no longer physically able to care for the ill family
member. The children cannot financially care for their own families if
they take time off work to care for their parent, nor do they have the
knowledge and nursing skills to do so. None of them wants their family
member to be admitted to a long-term care facility. However, after considering all possible solutions, they find that the best solution is placing
the family member in a long-term care facility.

Implement the Chosen Solution

After determining the best solution, implement it. Make sure all parties involved are informed appropriately. Keep in mind that change is
often difficult, and new issues may arise as the solution is implemented.
Address the issues appropriately and adequately, reexamining them in
light of the original problem.

Evaluate the Effectiveness of the Solution

Allow an adequate amount of time to pass after implementing the solution, then reevaluate the situation to determine the appropriateness
and effectiveness of the solution. Determine whether the root problem
has been solved or if the problem needs to be reevaluated.

*D*ECISION MAKING

Decision making is a process of using critical thinking in choosing the best option from several alternatives.

Clinical nurses are required to make efficient, sound, and effective decisions. **Decision making** is a process of using critical thinking in choosing the best option from several alternatives. The steps for decision making and problem solving are very similar, but decision making is different from problem solving. Decision making does not always solve the problem, but it supplies an immediate solution or action to a situation. Problem solving seeks to find a solution to the problem when the decisions have not solved the problem (Ham, 2002). The following example illustrates the difference between decision making and problem solving. A nursing student owns an older car that has prominent rust spots, uses a quart of oil a week, and has a hole in the tailpipe. At 9:00 one night, a bald tire goes flat. The student decides to call a friend to assist in changing the tire. After clinical at midnight a week later, the radiator overheats. The student again makes a decision, to call a friend for a ride home. After having made several decisions to address the situation, the student uses problem solving to review various options and decides to purchase a different car.

Many nursing decisions are based on the decision-making process. At first a nurse may make decisions slowly, working step-by-step through the decision-making process. Experienced nurses probably do not follow each step of the decision-making process as they make every decision; instead, by working through the steps to reach previous decisions they have developed critical thinking skills to complete the process quickly and effectively. The decision-making process may be used individually or in groups. Clinical nurses may use the process to solve a problem on the unit, such as scheduling or dispensing medications. When solving a group problem, communication through each step is vital for the success of the decision-making process.

Charts and Graphs for Decision Making

Several charts and graphs have been developed to assist in decision making. They include the decision tree, the Gantt chart, and the PERT (program evaluation and review technique) chart.

Decision Tree

The **decision tree** is a visual diagram of a decision, alternatives, risk factors, and possible outcomes. First, the decision regarding a problem is listed with at least two possible alternatives. The risk factors are listed for each alternative, followed by possible outcomes. It is called a tree because the diagram resembles one (see Figure 5–1). By working through the decision tree process, we recognize alternatives to a decision and the potential risks and consequences of each alternative decision (Tomey, 2000). Figure 5–2 is a completed decision tree using the earlier car example.

Gantt Chart

The **Gantt chart** is a grid schedule that allows you to see various tasks needed to complete a project. The chart consists of several columns, including one for the task, one for the person responsible for completing the task, and columns for the time frame for task completion (Figure 5–3). The time frame could be hours, days, months, or years. There is a separate row for each task or responsible person. A line is drawn in the time frame for tasks in progress. An X is placed on the completion point of the time frame. With a Gantt chart, you plan backward from the due date through the needed tasks.

PERT Chart

The **PERT chart** is a detailed graph of multiple tasks needing completion for a multitask project. The graph offers a diagram of projects needing completion before others can be started (Figure 5–4). This gives you a visual image of task sequencing. You provide time frames for task completion. The time frames can be broken down into shortest time, for completion with no complications, reasonable time, with usual complications, and longest time, with multiple complications (Tomey, 2000). These time frames are written on the lines between each task.

Using Gantt and PERT Charts

Gantt and PERT charts are used for decision making and for short- and long-term planning. When they are used in short- and long-term planning they assist with time management in detailed projects. They can

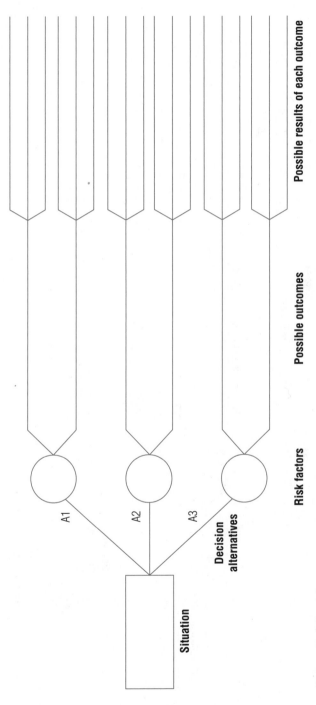

Figure 5–1 Decision tree.

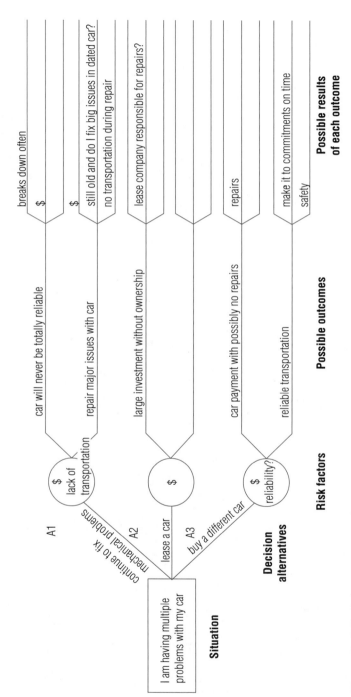

Figure 5–2 Decision tree example.

Task	Responsible person	Monday	Tuesday	Wednesday	Thursday	Friday

Figure 5–3 Gantt chart.

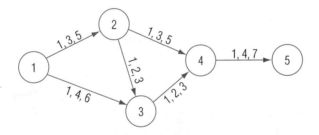

Figure 5–4 PERT chart. The numbers within the circles represent tasks to complete. In this PERT chart, task 1 needs completing before tasks 2 and 3, and task 2 slightly before 3. Tasks 1, 2, and 3 should be completed before task 4, and tasks 1, 2, 3, and 4 before task 5. The smaller numbers on each line represent possible time frames for completion of the task, with the first number being when the task could be completed most quickly, the second number most likely, and the last number the longest amount of time for completion. The arrows indicate the direction of task performance. Each of the numbers inside a circle represent an assigned task; for example, 1 = determine topic for research paper, 2 = obtain literature review.

help you in decision making and problem solving as you determine each step needed to make a decision, solve a problem, or complete a project. Sequencing tasks or steps in each of these charts develops critical thinking and decision-making skills. The charts also provide a visual method or process of decision making.

CRITICAL THINKING ACTIVITIES

1. Use a decision tree, Gantt chart, or PERT chart to work through a decision or plan a project, term paper, or committee responsibility. Draw the chart of your choice and compare your chart with your classmates.

2. Describe how you think your decision-making skills were developed by making the chart.

_____

_____

_____

$\mathscr{T}$HE NURSING PROCESS

The nursing process is a discipline-specific method used for decision making.

It is essential for nurses to make effective decisions in clinical practice. The **nursing process** is a discipline-specific method used for decision making. "The nursing process provides a logical and rational way for the nurse to solve problems and make decisions so the care given is appropriate and effective" (Hood & Leddy, 2003, p. 238). Even though the nursing process is a scientific, rational approach, it is carried out in a caring manner, truly making nursing a science and an art (Hood & Leddy).

The steps in the nursing process are assessment, nursing diagnosis, planning nursing care, implementing the plan, and evaluating the plan.

The steps in the nursing process are assessment, nursing diagnosis, planning nursing care, implementing the plan, and evaluating the plan. The client's condition frequently changes, resulting in the constant need to reassess, reevaluate, and revise the steps in the client's plan of care as developed through the nursing process. Therefore, these steps are not as linear as they may seem but are both integrated and circular in process (Figure 5–5).

Assessment

Assessment is obtaining a holistic view of a client by means of a thorough physical examination and a history collected through a personal therapeutic client interview, support system input, and a health record review. The assessment step includes data collection. The data collected is pertinent to planning and implementing client care. The primary source of data is the client, and secondary sources of data collection are the client's family members, other health personnel, and the client's medical records. The collected data is validated with other sources for accuracy and completeness.

Data is collected using various methods, including a body systems approach and Gordon's Functional Health Patterns (Gordon, 2002). These methods help to cluster the information for significance and relevance. Whatever method is used, the data pertains to nursing and nursing care.

Objective data is measurable and observable data obtained through a physical assessment. A therapeutic interview assists in obtaining subjective data from the client and includes the client's "feelings, perceptions, and concerns" (Delaune & Ladner, 2002, p. 96). Assessment is an ongoing process with each nurse-client interaction.

Nursing Diagnosis

As the data is collected, the nurse uses critical thinking to determine the relevance and pertinence of the information. She objectively analyzes the clustered data to see what it reveals about the client.

The nurse then develops a **nursing diagnosis** that is a statement describing the client's health problem. The nursing diagnosis consists of three parts: 1) the nursing diagnosis, 2) the etiologic phrase—the "related to" statement, and 3) the supporting signs and symptoms or defining charac-

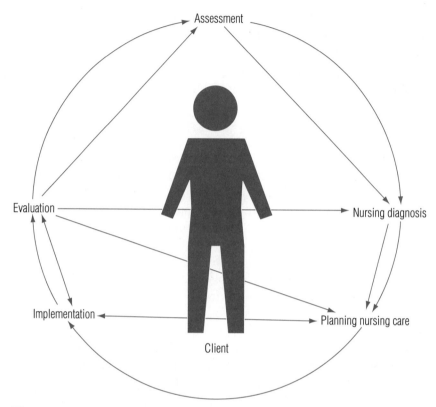

Figure 5–5 The nursing process is integrated and circular.

teristics. The nursing diagnosis is written according to the North American Nursing Diagnosis Association (NANDA) criteria. The nurse then collaborates with the client to develop goals for the expected outcomes of the nursing actions or implementation of the nursing plan of care. The nurse uses critical thinking and decision-making processes to develop the nursing diagnosis. Asking questions during this process is important because a valid appropriate, priority nursing diagnosis cannot be identified without considering all available data. See Table 5–1 for examples of critical thinking questions to ask during the nursing process.

Planning Nursing Care

In **planning nursing care,** the nurse writes client goals or objectives that address client needs and assist clients to an optimal health status. These goals determine the outcomes of the nursing care and are evaluated for degree of obtainment during the evaluation part of the nurs-

Table 5–1 Examples of critical-thinking questions for use with the nursing process

Assessment	Is the data complete? What other data do I need? What are some possible sources of the data? What assumptions or biases do I have in this situation? What is the client's point of view? Are there other points of view?
Diagnosis	What does the data mean? What else could be happening? Are there any gaps in the data? How are these data similar and how are they different? What assumptions or biases do I have in this situation? Have my assumptions affected my interpretation of the data? If so, in what way?
Outcome identification and planning	What are the goals for this client? What do I want to accomplish? How are my goals related to what the client wants to accomplish? What are the expected outcomes for this client? What interventions are to be used? Who is the best-qualified person to perform these interventions? How much involvement can the client and family or significant other have at this time? How much involvement does the client wish to have at this time?
Implementation	What is the client's current status? What are the most critical steps in this intervention? How must I alter the intervention to best meet this client's needs and maintain principles of safety? What is the client's response during and after the intervention? Is there a need to alter the intervention any way? If so, why and how?
Evaluation	Were the interventions successful in assisting the client to achieve the desired goals? How could things have been done differently? What data do I need to make new decisions? Where will I get the data? Were there assumptions, biases, or points of view that I missed that affected the outcomes? What can be done about these assumptions, biases, or points of view?

(From *Fundamentals of Nursing: Standards and Practice*, 2nd ed., by S. Delaune and P. Ladner, 2002, Clifton Park, NY: Thomson Delmar Learning.)

ing process. Ideally the nurse and client together determine the goals, "considering the client's capabilities, limitations, and desired lifestyle" (Hood & Leddy, 2003, p. 244).

Goals or expected outcomes are written in specific, measurable, time-limited, and realistic terms so that they can be evaluated objectively once the nursing interventions have been implemented. **Nursing**

interventions are the nursing care or activities done to and with the client to obtain the goal of optimum health. Nursing interventions change as the client's condition changes.

Implementing the Plan

Implementing the plan is the nurse's completion of interventions to assist the client to an optimum health state or a quality end of life. Nursing actions assist the client in reaching optimum health goals. Nursing actions require nursing skills, teaching, communication, and collaboration with various health personnel. "Interventions are carried out with sensitivity to the client's feelings and are based on the client's individuality" (Hood & Leddy, 2003, p. 248). It is important to record the client's condition, specific nursing interventions or nursing actions performed and the client's response to the interventions, and client outcomes (Delaune & Ladner, 2002).

Evaluating the Plan

The cognitive processes of the nursing process are the true form of nursing as a science, and the caring nursing interventions are the art of nursing.

When **evaluating** the plan, the nurse reviews the client's progress toward the stated goals. The goals are evaluated as goals met, partially met, or not met. The evaluation phase of the nursing process is continuous and ongoing. Depending on the results of the evaluation, the nurse will reassess the client for goal attainment, reprioritize the problems, develop new goals, and revise the nursing interventions. If the goals were met, the nurse-client relationship may cease. Each phase of the nursing process is recorded on the client's record.

We have presented the steps in a linear form, but the nursing process is interrelated and interdependent in each phase. The cognitive processes of the nursing process are the true form of nursing as a science, and the caring nursing interventions are the art of nursing.

𝒜PPLICATION

The LPN's role in the nursing process is collecting data, documenting that data, relating the data to the RN, and contributing suggestions to the care plans regarding clients' identified needs. The RN facilitates and oversees the nursing process. She initiates the plan of care by delegating responsibilities to team members according to responsibility and capability levels; for example, aides bathe and weigh the client and LPNs collect assessment data. The RN performs a complete, thorough assessment by physically assessing the client, interviewing the client, and referring to multiple sources for client information. Together, the RN, the client, and other health care team members set goals for the client's return to a maximum health state. The RN then determines appropriate nursing interventions to address the client's individual health needs. The LPN completes nursing interventions according to the stated nurse practice act. As the nursing interventions are implemented, the RN, with the LPN's input, determines whether the nursing goals/outcomes are being met. If the nursing interventions are not accomplishing the client's goals/outcomes, the RN, with input from the LPN, determines nursing interventions that will meet the goals/outcomes. If the client's condition changes so that the goals/outcomes are not realistic, the RN rewrites the goals/outcomes and proceeds through the nursing process steps as needed.

CRITICAL THINKING ACTIVITY

1. Using the scenario at the beginning of this chapter, develop a plan of care using the steps of the nursing process.

   • Assessment:

   _____

   _____

   _____

   • Nursing diagnosis:

   _____

   _____

   _____

- Plan nursing care (client goals):

_____

_____

_____

- Implement the plan (nursing actions):

_____

_____

_____

- Evaluate the plan:

_____

_____

_____

Table 5–2 Comparing the steps of problem solving, decision-making, and the nursing process

Problem Solving	Decision Making	Nursing Process
Identify the problem	Address the problem	Assess client needs
Generate possible solutions and examine suggested solutions	Consider the options	Decide on appropriate nursing diagnosis
Choose the best solution	Choose a solution	Plan nursing care
Implement the chosen solution	Implement the choice	Implement nursing action
Evaluate the effectiveness of the solution for the problem and decide if the problem has been resolved	Evaluate the outcome	Evaluate the outcomes

(Revised from Tomey, 2000.)

SUMMARY

Benner et al. (1996) support using intuition based on facts in clinical decision making. The decision-making process is similar to the problem-solving process and the nursing process (see Table 5–2). Each of these processes takes a scientific problem-solving approach. In problem solving, the problem is analyzed thoroughly and multiple solutions or options are reviewed before a decision is made and implemented. Decision making requires critical thinking to choose the best option for the directed action. The nursing process is the nurse's systematic method of clinical decision making.

Sometimes students find working through the nursing process very rigorous, time consuming, and laborious. Yet the nursing process is one method, or process, of developing expert clinical decision-making skills.

Nurses making sound decisions provide quality care to clients. Effective, sound decisions are needed to conserve time, resources, and energy. Develop your critical thinking skills and your decision-making and problem-solving abilities so that you will soon be the facilitator of the nursing process, providing quality care to the client.

𝒞HAPTER REFLECTIONS

1. Where would you place Tameka in Benner et al.'s five-stage novice-to-expert practice model?

2. What skills did Tameka use when she decided to seek advice from a more experienced co-worker?

3. If you were in Tameka's position, would you view yourself as an incompetent nurse? Would this be an appropriate reaction to the situation? Why or why not?

4. Using each of the decision-making steps presented in this chapter, what would you do to address Tameka's client scenario?

REFERENCES

Benner, P., Tanner, C., & Chesla, C. (1996). *Expertise in nursing practice: Caring, clinical judgment, and ethics.* New York: Springer.

Delaune, S., & Ladner, P. (2002). *Fundamentals of nursing: Standards and practice* (2nd ed.). Clifton Park, NY: Thomson Delmar Learning.

Gordon, M. (2002). *Manual of nursing diagnosis* (10th ed.). St. Louis, MO: Mosby.

Ham, K. (2002). *From LPN to RN: Role transitions.* Philadelphia: W. B. Saunders.

Hood, L., & Leddy, S. (2003). *Leddy and Pepper's conceptual bases of professional nursing* (5th ed.). Philadelphia: Lippincott Williams & Wilkins.

Tomey, A. (2000). *Guide to nursing management and leadership* (6th ed.). St. Louis, MO: Mosby.

SUGGESTED RESOURCES

Gregory, K. (2000). *Nurse the patient! Medical Economics Inc.* [On-line]. Available: http://80-proquest.umi.com.fortway

O'Reilly, P. (1993). *Barriers to effective clinical decision making in nursing* [On-line]. Available: http://www.clininfo.health.nsw.gov.au/hospolic/stvincents/1993/a04.html

Pesut, D., & Herman, J. (1999). *Clinical reasoning: The art and science of critical and creative thinking.* Clifton Park, NY: Thomson Delmar Learning.

Chapter 6
Client Teaching

▼ ▼ ▼ ▼ ▼ ▼ ▼

LEARNING OBJECTIVES

By the end of this chapter, you should be able to:

1. Explain the role of the nurse as teacher.
2. List the principles of adult learning.
3. List factors that interfere with learning.
4. Develop a client teaching plan.

KEY TERMS

Andragogy
Pedagogy
Teach
Teaching-learning

SCENARIO

Carlos, an LPN for one year, has been asked by his RN mentor to complete the discharge teaching plan for his assigned client. He completes the discharge instructions by filling in information in the appropriate sections as guided by the form. He returns to the RN to see if the discharge information is accurate and complete. Carlos relies on the RN for the final decision about implementing the discharge teaching according to hospital policy.

THINK ABOUT IT

1. Compare your client teaching experience with Carlos's.
2. How do facility policies affect your ability to complete client teaching?

*I*NTRODUCTION

Because clients are quickly discharged from the hospital and often are expected to continue complex care, teaching is essential to effective health care.

In a recent research study entitled "A Study of Professional Nurses' Perceptions of Patient Education," 92 percent of the nurses stated that client teaching was "a priority in their nursing care" (Marcum, Ridenour, Shaff, Hammons, & Taylor, 2002, p. 112). The teaching-learning process can be informal or formal. A nurse can teach informally by explaining the action of heparin when giving a heparin injection. Formal teaching usually includes some preparation of a teaching plan to explain a concept to a client, such as preoperative preparation for surgery, diabetic diet instruction, and self-administration of insulin. Because clients are quickly discharged from the hospital and often are expected to continue complex care, teaching is essential to effective health care.

In this chapter we will discuss the nurse as a teacher, principles of adult learning, factors that interfere with teaching-learning situations, and effective methods of teaching clients. You will have an opportunity to develop a teaching plan for a client applying the teaching-learning principles presented in the following pages.

*T*HE NURSE AS TEACHER

Teaching is an integral part of nursing. Sandra Cornett (2003) effectively stated the emotional, tangible, and intangible components of teaching when she said, "Teaching is the part of caring that stays with a patient and his or her family long after all physical contact has stopped. The impact of teaching is often delayed and the results are usually not seen by the health care provider while the patient is in the hospital" (p. 1). When a nurse teaches, there are lasting implications.

CRITICAL THINKING ACTIVITY

1. Write two concepts that someone taught you in the past and that you are still able to recall.

_____

_____

_____

2. How long has it been since you were taught these concepts?

_____

_____

_____

Nurses not only teach clients, they also teach students and model nursing care for students. These nurses set standards for the next generation of nurses. It is important that nurses be exemplary in their ethical choices, client care, and professional standards. This role modeling is an honor and a responsibility for the nurse. Even though nurses are very involved in teaching students, the rest of this chapter will address the nurse as client teacher.

CRITICAL THINKING ACTIVITY

1. List two nurses who have served as your teaching role models. Relate your reasons for choosing these nurses.

_____

_____

_____

_____

Teaching Defined

Every nurse-client interaction is a potential teaching-learning opportunity.

Nurses are the key educators in health care. To **teach** is to effectively share information so that another can learn. The goal of client teaching is to increase knowledge, impart skills, and change behavior. Teaching assists the client in coping with future events related to his condition. Teaching is not restricted to caring for the present condition, but it also includes information to promote a healthy lifestyle. Every nurse-client interaction is a potential teaching-learning opportunity. In these interactions, both the nurse and the client can learn from each other.

Informal Teaching

Effective teaching can be completed in an efficient, timely manner. As nurses do daily activities, such as ambulating and bathing clients, administering medications, and changing dressings, they can use these opportunities to educate the clients about ambulation techniques, stimulation of circulation with bathing, medication actions and side effects, and dressing-changing procedures. Every interaction can be used to improve the client's knowledge of his condition. Teaching clients about tests, procedures, and surgery are other educational opportunities.

CRITICAL THINKING ACTIVITY

1. Relate something you taught a client. What method did you use to teach the client?

_____

_____

_____

Clients in health care settings are more educated than they were a few years ago because of their use of the Internet and other information that is available to them within their homes. Clients' familiarity with computers offers other effective teaching methods besides one-on-one nurse-client interaction. Independent study worksheets or booklets, videos, and computer instruction can assist the nurse in relaying valuable information to the client.

Formal Teaching

It is important to listen to what the client and his family say about the information taught to accurately assess the client and family's comprehension.

Client teaching is not always done informally but can also be very effective in structured teaching-learning situations. In a structured setting, a nurse selects specific content to teach a client and writes specific client-oriented goals for the teaching-learning session. The nurse plans the session content and prepares specific effective methods of communicating the information. After the session the nurse evaluates the content, presentation, and methods. The nurse and client each should be given an opportunity to evaluate the teaching-learning session.

Chronic illnesses are challenging experiences for clients. By teaching the client about the disease and methods of handling the disease, the nurse assists him in making necessary life changes to deal with the disease condition. The nurse can also suggest changes to accommodate client care within the home. These suggestions include shower grab bars, elevated toilet seats, and adaptive handles for kitchen utensils. Self-management is the teaching goal for clients with chronic illness (Cornett, 2003).

It is important to listen to what the client and the family say about the information taught to accurately assess the client and family's comprehension. If the nurse has the client repeat the instructions, he can reteach or clarify misconceptions as needed.

PRINCIPLES OF ADULT LEARNING

Literature supports the theory that adults learn differently than children. Knowles (1980) coined the term **andragogy,** "the art and science of helping adults learn" as opposed to the commonly known term *pedagogy,* "the art and science of teaching children" (p. 43). Knowles was one of the first persons to propose adult learning principles. Lawler (1991) expanded on Knowles's principles and suggested nine principles of adult learning. Lawler's nine principles of adult learning are:

1. Adults learn best in an environment of mutual respect.
2. Adults like a collaborative style of learning.
3. Adults' educational knowledge builds on life experiences.
4. Adult education should encourage insightful critical thinking.
5. Adults learn from problem-solving situation scenarios.
6. Adults take pleasure in applying their learning in real-life situations.
7. Adults enjoy participating in the learning environment by identifying personal learning needs.
8. Adult learners are empowered through education.
9. Adult education provides and encourages self-directed and independent learning.

Lawler's principles apply in teaching-learning environments such as adult educational settings. Pamela Schuster (2000) also has developed four adult learning principles, but she has applied them more directly to client teaching situations. Schuster's four adult learning principles as they relate to client teaching are:

1. Build on previous experiences.
2. Focus on immediate concerns first.
3. Adapt teaching to lifestyle.
4. Make [the client] an active participant. (pp. 214–216)

Let's discuss teaching concepts that we can glean from these adult learning principles by Lawler and Schuster.

Develop a Climate of Trust

To provide the best client-learning environment, the nurse needs to personally respect the client and the client's learning desires.

It is important for the nurse to encourage and develop a climate of trust and respect with the client. To provide the best client-learning environment, the nurse needs to personally respect the client and the client's learning desires. It is important for the nurse to communicate confidence in the client's ability to learn the material verbally and nonverbally (Hood & Leddy, 2003). The client also needs to trust and respect the nurse. An informal and relaxed atmosphere provides an environment conducive for teaching-learning. By being open, honest, and truly interested in the client's concerns, the nurse can encourage an effective, trusting, teaching-learning environment.

Encourage Participation

Encourage the client to list and prioritize learning goals. The written learning goals provide a visual plan of action for both nurse and client. The written goals also provide a record to evaluate progress and achievement. Both client and nurse can have a sense of accomplishment as the learning goals are achieved.

Build on Past Experiences

To build on past experiences, Schuster (2000) suggests that we determine what the client knows about the subject being taught. Once the client's knowledge base is determined, we can build from that point. It is important to ascertain the client's past experience with health, illness, health care, or the behaviors we would like the client to change. How a client thinks about these concepts will affect what and how we teach. It will also allow us to address the client's fears or misconceptions about these concepts. The client may need to unlearn incorrect information and relearn new information and techniques. This sequence of steps is part of the unfreezing stage of the change process discussed in Chapter 2. An example of relearning as it relates to the change process is a client who had surgery 10 years ago and was given pain medication by the nurse. He is now being hospitalized and during his preoperative teaching is told that he now participates in controlling his pain. After surgery, he will press a button on a patient-controlled analgesia (PCA) pump to receive a small dose of pain medication through his IV without the assistance of the nurse. He then can press the button any time he is experiencing pain. In this situation, the client has to relearn the way to receive pain relief: that he does not have to call a nurse for pain medication but can press a button to control his postoperative pain.

CRITICAL THINKING ACTIVITIES

1. Think of an experience in your life that has occurred more than once and describe how it was different the second time.

   _____

   _____

   _____

2. As an LPN-RN student, do you think you will need to unlearn some nursing concepts previously taught?

   _____

   _____

   _____

3. How can you use your experience of learning to help your clients build on their past experiences?

_____

_____

_____

Address Immediate Concerns

Adults want information for their immediate concerns. The client may have a more pressing and different concern than the nurse. If a client is worried about children at home that may lack supervision, that need must be met before the client can concentrate on learning how to lower his blood pressure. The nurse must use the therapeutic skills of active listening, clarifying, and summarizing to determine and address the client's concerns before teaching methods for lowering blood pressure.

Assist in Lifestyle Adjustments

Our teaching needs to assist the client in making lifestyle adjustments. For example, if a client works long hours we need to offer suggestions and assist him in finding ways to fit an exercise routine into his schedule. These suggestions could include taking a walk at lunch, stopping by a gym on the way to or from work, or purchasing a treadmill or stationary bicycle to use when watching television.

Involvement in the Learning Process

Clients learn quicker and retain the information longer if they are actively involved in the learning process.

Adult learners like to determine their learning needs and be involved in the learning process. Teaching methods that enhance client involvement are discussion, demonstration with return demonstration, and scenarios with problem-solving situations. These scenarios relate lifelike situations with questions stimulating the client to analyze lifelike responses. For example, if the nurse is teaching diabetic classes, he could demonstrate insulin administration and ask the client to do a return demonstration. The nurse provides immediate positive reinforcement when the client performs the return demonstration correctly. A problem scenario could be provided by asking the client how to handle insulin administration correctly if he has the flu. This discussion gives the client an opportunity to gain confidence that he will handle the situation appropriately when it arises outside the teaching environment. These methods are often more effective than lecture and provide an opportunity to verify whether learning has occurred and whether we have communicated effectively. Offering the client an opportunity to evaluate the teaching-learning experience provides feedback for the nurse to improve his teaching techniques.

Following the described teaching-learning principles enables and gives power to the client. It equips the client to successfully manage individual health concerns and issues.

CRITICAL THINKING ACTIVITY

1. Think of a time you utilized one of the adult learning principles when you were teaching a client. Write about the experience.

_____

_____

_____

_____

_____

*I*NTERFERING FACTORS

In a study by Marcum et al. (2002), nurses listed the three main factors that interfered with client education as time, staffing, and client receptiveness. The three factors the nurses identified that could assist them in client teaching were more time to teach, teaching guidance sheets, and available resources. The nursing shortage and client assignment load definitely affect the available time a nurse has to teach clients. One thing that could assist both the time factor for the nurse and staffing issues is providing basic teaching sheets that could be regularly used in the facility, for example, information on medications frequently dispensed, information on common diagnoses, and basic discharge instructions. In this way, a nurse could quickly pick up a pamphlet and share it with a client even on a very busy day. Some hospital units provide access to a library, a computer, or videos, so the client can research health information as desired. Providing these resources would free the

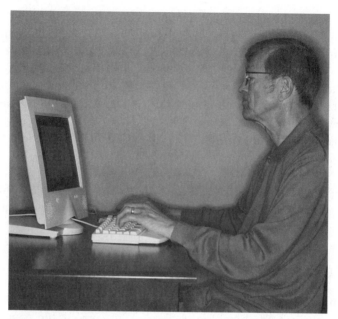

Figure 6–1 Encourage clients to use a computer to research health information. (Courtesy of PhotoDisc.)

nurse for other responsibilities and would be a vital educational tool for the client teaching-learning process (Figure 6–1).

Clients' emotional and/or physiological state, lifestyle, or value system may affect their receptiveness to what we would like to teach them. Anxiety about a diagnosis may decrease teaching receptivity. Older clients may have memory problems or take a passive role during the teaching session, especially if their children are present. Before we start teaching a client, it is important to assess his or her openness to being taught (Figure 6–2).

In *Communication: The Key to the Therapeutic Relationship*, Schuster (2000) lists four factors that interfere with learning. These factors are emotional state, physiological issues, defense mechanisms, and cultural and value complexities.

Emotional State

Before beginning a teaching session, assess the client's emotional state. If the client is anxious about his condition, his anxiety will interfere

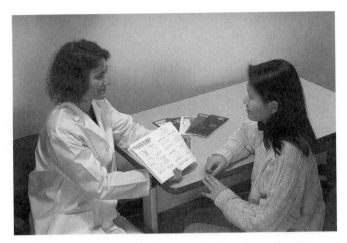

Figure 6–2 Printed resources can assist with client teaching.

Emotional state
Physiological issues
Defense mechanisms
Cultural and value complexities

Box 6–1 Factors that interfere with learning

with his openness to what is being taught. Perhaps the client is grieving over the loss of a limb or limitations of the disease that will change his lifestyle. These emotions will definitely affect the client's ability and desire to comprehend what you are teaching. By first addressing the emotional state with therapeutic communication techniques, you may open the client to being taught small segments of material at separate intervals. This decreases his need to concentrate for longer periods of time. The client may want to learn what is taught but simply be unable to concentrate for long periods.

Physiological Issues

If a client is hungry, tired, nauseated, or in pain, it would be best to do teaching at a different time. Some clients may hesitate to tell you how they are feeling. Others may ask you to return at a different time because they would like to understand what you have to teach but are not able to concentrate at that time. It is important to assess the client's physiological state to determine the best teaching moment.

Defense Mechanisms

A client who needs to make a lifestyle change because of a particular disease may not be ready to make the needed change and may put up barriers or make excuses not to change. An example is a client with an elevated cholesterol level. The client may not be ready to make the needed diet, exercise, or medication changes. He makes excuses for why the new diet will not work or denies the need to exercise because a friend with the same problem lived to old age without exercising. You need to continue to develop a relationship of trust and educate the client about the disease until he sees the need for and desires to make the change. Also, you can assist the client by discussing possible ways his present lifestyle could change to accommodate the needed diet and exercise changes.

Cultural and Value Complexities

A client's culture or value system may present barriers to teaching. For example, a client with a heart disease who likes high-fat foods may find it difficult to adjust to the decreased fat content in the diet. You need to consider the client's culture and assist him with menu modifications to accommodate his physical condition.

CRITICAL THINKING ACTIVITY

1. Write down an example of one interfering factor you have seen in providing client care.

   _____

   _____

   _____

CLIENT TEACHING

We are potentially changed with each interaction we have with others and, therefore, have the opportunity to perceive our world differently and change our behavior.

Hood and Leddy (2003) define the **teaching-learning** process as "an interpersonal process in which both the teacher and the learner acquire new information, experience new relatedness, and behave in new ways as a result of the relationship" (p. 485). Often we think of the teaching-learning process as conveying information to the learner and forget the fact that we as nurses learn significant information from the clients we teach. Some information we learn from our nurse-client interactions is how to better phrase our teaching statements, what type of teaching works and what does not work with the client, and what to include in the teaching plan. We are potentially changed with each interaction we have with others and, therefore, have the opportunity to perceive our world differently and change our behavior.

At the beginning of this chapter, we discussed how we could teach when walking a client or changing a dressing. This is an informal process of teaching clients. The formal teaching process includes writing teaching objectives/goals, planning teaching content, implementing the teaching plan, and evaluating the teaching process. The nursing process and the teaching process use the same steps: assessment, planning, implementation, and evaluation, as shown in Table 6–1.

Assessment

First, we assess the client's teaching needs. We determine the client's knowledge base by asking questions. What does the client know about the disease condition? What does he know about treating the condition? What does he know about the prescribed medications? Is a diet change required? Does the client need special equipment? Does the client know

Table 6–1 Comparison of nursing process and teaching process

	Nursing Process	Teaching Process
Assessment	Client physical, psychosocial, spiritual, and cultural needs	Client knowledge base Client teaching-learning needs
Planning	Goals to achieve or maintain optimum health	Goals to achieve teaching-learning needs
Implementation	Nursing actions to meet client's needs	Teaching plan to meet client's learning needs
Evaluation	Attainment of client goals/outcomes	Attainment of educational goals and learning objectives

how to operate the equipment? Once we determine the client's knowledge base, we decide what further information the client needs to obtain optimum health. Keep in mind that a client's last grade completed in school does not always indicate his comprehension or knowledge level.

What does the client know about the disease condition?
What does the client know about treating the condition?
What does the client know about the prescribed medications?
Is a diet change required?
Does the client need special equipment?
Does the client know how to operate the equipment?

Box 6–2 Questions to ask to determine the client's teaching needs

Planning

To change a client's behavior we must teach to three domains: cognitive domain (knowledge), affective domain (emotions), and psychomotor domain (application or behavior change) (Bloom, 1956).

After assessment, the next step is planning. We plan what we need to teach the client, writing down client objectives or learning goals. It is important for the nurse to obtain input from the client as to what he desires to learn.

As we first start formal teaching plans, it is important to make the teaching plan simple and preferable to teach only one concept, such as information about the disease, or medications, or changing a dressing. If the teaching plan has multiple subjects, the client may learn and retain more information if the teaching sessions are short and one segment of information is taught at a time.

To change a client's behavior we must teach to three domains: cognitive domain (knowledge), affective domain (emotions), and psychomotor domain (application or behavior change) (Bloom, 1956). When preparing a teaching plan, write a goal for each of the domains. An easy way to write a goal for each domain is to remember the words *know* (knowledge), *feel/desire* (emotions), and *do* (application/action). Know addresses the knowledge level and would translate to the nursing process as a nursing diagnosis of "knowledge deficit. . . ." Feel/desire activates the emotions. And do results in application and action. If you were teaching about medications, your goals could be:

1. The client will state (know) the actions, administration times, side effects, and special considerations when taking the medications.
2. The client will express a desire (feel/desire) to learn the described information about medications.
3. The client will take and explain (do) the medication actions, administration times, side effects, and special considerations.

These goals are written in realistic, specific, measurable terms so they can easily be evaluated.

Myrna Spicer (2003) suggests writing one educational goal and then listing other, related learning objectives under the educational goal. This works very well if you are teaching complex material. The educational goal is written in broad terms, then learning objectives are written in specific, action-oriented terms to reach the main goal. When writing learning objectives, attach action verbs to the knowledge or skill statement desired of the client. Let's examine an educational goal and learning objectives when teaching a client a cardiac lifestyle change. Refer to Box 6–3 for an example.

Educational goal

The client will learn how to live a healthy lifestyle to avoid cardiac complications.

Action-oriented objectives

List	factors that contribute to heart disease
List	foods low in fat
List	foods low in sodium
Develop	a low-fat, low-sodium diet
Describe	an exercise program to reduce cardiac complications (Spicer, 2003)
Discuss	present lifestyle factors that may lead to heart disease

---

Box 6–3 Example of one type of teaching plan

The goals should be written so that each individual health care provider can interpret them exactly the same. The more specific, realistic, and measurable the terms used in writing the goals, the easier it will be to evaluate whether the goals have been met.

Implementation

The third step in the teaching process is implementation. The nurse researches content material to meet the cognitive goal. An example is a nurse researching information about medication actions, times of administration, side effects, and special considerations in taking the medication. This information is written down so that the client can refer to the material as needed. Prepared instruction sheets are great tools for client teaching. Nurses and clients both benefit. Nurses should be able to access the instruction sheets easily so that they can use them in client teaching. The client will receive all the needed information, and important items will not be omitted.

If teaching is done in a structured setting, the teaching session can include three sections: introduction, body, and conclusion (Cornett, 2003). During the introduction the teacher introduces himself to the client, explains the purpose of the teaching session, and lists the expected outcomes. The client is included in setting goals for the teaching-learning session. In the body of the teaching session, the information is presented with as much client involvement as possible. Handouts, videos, computer instruction, or other teaching materials are offered. In the conclusion, the client is asked to do or perform the expected outcomes. When the client lists information or does a return demonstration, it is important for the teacher to give positive feedback to the client (Cornett).

Evaluation

> *To evaluate the teaching-learning session and client knowledge, make sure each teaching goal was completed.*

To evaluate the teaching-learning session and client knowledge, check to see if each of the teaching goals was completed. If the goals are written in specific, measurable terms, the evaluation should be completed rather easily. Evaluate whether the teaching methods and content were appropriate. Could more effective methods have been used? Does the content need to be presented in a different order? Include client feedback on the teaching-learning session. The evaluation process will guide the revision of the next teaching-learning session. What needs to be retaught to the client? What new teaching does the client need?

APPLICATION

An example of a teaching plan using the concepts presented in this chapter appears in Box 6–4. Review that example and then, using it as a model, use Box 6–5 to create a teaching plan from your own clinical experience with a client.

Scenario: Lorenzo was admitted to the medical unit with a deep vein thrombosis in his right leg. He has responded well to the heparin drip and has transitioned to Coumadin. He is now ready to be dismissed on Coumadin. The physician has asked the student nurse to teach Lorenzo about the action, side effects, needed laboratory appointments, and dietary precautions for Coumadin. Because this is the first time the student has taught a client about a medication, he asks his professor for assistance. The professor offers a teaching-plan sample to the student, who then proceeds to write the following teaching plan.

Assessment

Knowledge base of client:

Lorenzo has an associate degree from a local community college.

Past experiences with health, illness, health care, and lifestyle:

Lorenzo works on the assembly line at a major car manufacturing plant. He states he generally is healthy and has only had the flu twice in his life. He has regular dental checkups and yearly physical exams. This is the first time he has had a clot.

Interfering factors: emotional, physical, defense mechanisms, cultural and value complexities:

Lorenzo has had several friends visit him in the hospital. He is fairly active and enjoys working on cars in the evening and weekends. He states that he is concerned about how being on Coumadin will affect his lifestyle.

Box 6–4 Teaching plan example

He wants to know if he will be able to work on cars and drink beer while watching ballgames with his friends.

Questions to ask this individual client to determine knowledge base:

1. Describe what you do at work.
2. What do you know about how clots form?
3. What are the complications of having a clot?
4. Do you know any methods to prevent clot formation?
5. What do you know about Coumadin?

Planning

Bloom's goal-writing method

Client's learning goals:

Lorenzo will describe the action, list the side effects, explain the importance of regular laboratory appointments, and state dietary changes relating to Coumadin.

Write a goal to each domain: cognitive, affective, and psychomotor:

Cognitive: State the action, list the side effects, explain the importance of regular laboratory appointments, and state dietary changes relating to Coumadin.

Affective: Express a desire to make the lifestyle adjustments of taking Coumadin.

Psychomotor: Take Coumadin at the correct times, observing for side effects, with regular lab appointments, and following dietary specifications.

Spicer's educational goal and learning objectives method

Educational goal:

Lorenzo will learn how to safely take Coumadin.

Box 6–4 (continued)

Learning objectives:

Action verb   *Desired knowledge/skill*

List   the action of Coumadin
List   the side effects of Coumadin
Describe   the rationale for regular laboratory appointments
State   the normal INR level
List   dietary specifications while on Coumadin

Implementation

In outline form, complete the teaching information for each section: introduction, body, and conclusion. List the method that you will use for each teaching item. List supplies and equipment needed to teach the content adequately using the chosen method.

Introduction

Information to teach:

Introduction of self:

Hello. I am _____ and I am a student nurse.

Purpose of teaching session:

Your physician has asked that I explain how you can safely and effectively take Coumadin.

Expected outcomes:

At the end of our discussion you will state the action of Coumadin, be able to list some side effects of Coumadin, state the importance of maintaining regular laboratory appointments, and list specific dietary considerations.

Review client goals for the teaching-learning session:

Is there anything else you would like to know about taking Coumadin?

Box 6–4 (continued)

Teaching method:

Discussion

Client involvement:

Give the client time to think of other information he would like to know about taking Coumadin.

Supplies/equipment needed:

Goals of the teaching session written for the client.

Body

Information to teach:

Outline of teaching information:

The clot may have formed in your leg because of standing in one spot for an extended period. Perhaps you could flex your leg at times and exercise your legs as much as possible while working on the assembly line.

Coumadin is an anticoagulant. That means it prevents blood from clotting.

Every medication has some side effects. Coumadin causes you to bleed and bruise easily. Notify your doctor if you notice blood when you brush your teeth, urinate, or defecate, or if you have a nose bleed. Your Coumadin dose may need to be reevaluated.

It is important for you to have a lab test called an INR drawn on a regular basis. It will be drawn more frequently at first and then on a regular basis once the Coumadin dose is regulated.

The normal desired INR for a person on Coumadin who has had a clot is 2–3. The Coumadin dose is regulated according to the level of the INR.

When you are taking Coumadin, you should avoid foods high in vitamin K. These foods are the dark green vegetables like spinach, cabbage, brussels sprouts, and broccoli. Alcohol also has an anticoagulant effect so excessive amounts of alcohol should be avoided. If you eat broccoli twice a week and have one beer a week, then continue as you presently are eating. Just do not eat broccoli three times in one day.

Box 6–4 (continued)

Maintain a somewhat routine diet of green leafy vegetables and moderate alcohol consumption.

Teaching method:

Discussion and question and answer with client.
Review brochure on Coumadin.

Client involvement:

Question and answer with client.
Review brochure with client.
Discuss regular eating habits with client.

Supplies/equipment needed:

Brochure on Coumadin

Conclusion

Information to teach:

What is the client to do or perform?

1. State the action of Coumadin.

2. List the side effects of Coumadin.

3. State the importance of maintaining regular laboratory appointments.

4. List specific dietary considerations.

Nurse's positive feedback to the client:

Give Lorenzo positive feedback on information he has learned.
Correct any information that he has not understood.
Ask if he has any questions.

Teaching method:

Question and answer

Client involvement:

Have the client complete each teaching objective.

Box 6–4 (continued)

Supplies/equipment needed:

N/A

Evaluation

Were the learning objectives achieved?
What would have improved this teaching-learning session?
What worked?
What did not work as well as desired?
What could have been included?
What could have been deleted?
Could more effective teaching methods have been used?
Did the content sequence need rearranging?
What did the client think of the teaching-learning session?
How did I facilitate or enhance communication in the teaching-learning session?
Did anything interfere or block communication in the teaching-learning session?

Reconstruct the needed teaching:

What needs to be re-taught to the client?
What new teaching does the client need?

Box 6–4 (continued)

Now refer to Box 6–5 and create your own teaching plan.

Assessment

Knowledge base of client:

Past experiences with health, illness, health care, and lifestyle:

Interfering factors: emotional, physical, defense mechanisms, cultural and value complexities:

Questions to ask this individual client to determine knowledge base:

1.

2.

3.

4.

5.

Box 6–5 Create your own teaching plan

Planning

Bloom's goal-writing method
Client's learning goals:

Write a goal for each domain: cognitive, affective, and psychomotor:

Cognitive:

Affective:

Psychomotor:

Spicer's educational goal and learning objectives method

Educational goal:
Learning objectives:

Action verb   *Desired knowledge/skill*

Box 6–5 (continued)

Implementation

In outline form, complete the teaching information for each section: introduction, body, and conclusion. List the method that you will use for each teaching item. List supplies and equipment needed to teach the content adequately using the chosen method.

Introduction

Information to teach:

Introduction of self:

Purpose of teaching session:

Expected outcomes:

Review client goals for teaching-learning session:

Box 6–5 (continued)

Teaching method:

Client involvement:

Supplies/equipment needed:

Body

Information to teach:

Outline of teaching information:

Teaching method:

Client involvement:

Box 6–5 (continued)

Supplies/equipment needed:

Conclusion

Information to teach:

What is the client to do or perform?

Nurse's positive feedback to the client:

Teaching method:

Client involvement:

Supplies/equipment needed:

Box 6–5 (continued)

Evaluation

Were the learning objectives obtained?
What would have improved this teaching-learning session?
What worked?
What did not work as well as desired?
What could have been included?
What could have been deleted?
Could more effective methods have been used?
Did the content sequence need rearranging?
What did the client think of the teaching-learning session?

Reconstruct the needed teaching:

What needs to be retaught to the client?

What new teaching does the client need?

Box 6–5 (continued)

SUMMARY

Teaching is a vital part of health care. In this chapter we have reviewed adult learning principles, factors that interfere with learning, and specific techniques to improve client teaching-learning sessions. You were guided through the development of a teaching plan.

As an LPN you have played a vital role in the client teaching process. You participated in the client teaching role by gathering data, identifying client teaching needs, and reporting the information to the RN. You also may have taught some basic information to the client.

Now, as you become an RN, you can expect to play a larger role in client teaching. As an RN you will be expected to do thorough assessments, finding any factors that interfere with or enhance client teaching and to develop the most appropriate method of client education. The RN usually oversees and coordinates the client's teaching care plans and reviews and coordinates discharge-teaching plans. Not only does the RN do client teaching, he also completes client family teaching, staff education, and participates in unit continuing education. RNs may also be involved in client teaching positions such as staff education, diabetic teaching, and organ procurement.

You have tools to impart needed information to your clients in a new role. Now is your opportunity to improve nursing care by putting these principles into nursing practice.

CHAPTER REFLECTIONS

1. After reading this chapter, how will you change your client teaching experiences?
2. Obviously not all the teaching you do will require a teaching plan as described in this chapter, but if you use a teaching plan, how will it affect your client teaching?
3. How did working through the teaching plan and teaching a client change your approach, attitude, or ideas about client teaching?

REFERENCES

Anderson, L., & Krathwohl, D. (2001). *A taxonomy for learning, teaching and assessing: A revision of Bloom's taxonomy of educational objectives.* New York: Longman.

Cornett, S. (2003). *Principles for patient teaching* [On-line]. Available: http://devweb3.vip.ohio-state.edu/Materials/PDFDocs/principles-teach.pdf

Hood, L., & Leddy, S. (2003). *Leddy and Pepper's conceptual bases of professional nursing* (5th ed.). Philadelphia: Lippincott Williams & Wilkins.

Knowles, M. (1980). *The modern practice of adult education: From pedagogy to andragogy.* Chicago: Follett.

Lawler, P. (1991). *The keys to adult learning: Theory and practical strategies.* Philadelphia: Research for Better Schools.

Marcum, J., Ridenour, M., Shaff, G., Hammons, M., & Taylor, M. (2002). A study of professional nurses' perceptions of patient education. *Journal of Continuing Education in Nursing, 33*(3), 112–118.

Schuster, P. (2000). *Communication: The key to the therapeutic relationship.* Philadelphia: F.A. Davis.

Spicer, M. (2003). *How to design and use a patient teaching module* [On-line]. Available: http://www.PubMed.com

SUGGESTED RESOURCES

Barber-Parker, E. (2002). Integrating patient teaching into bedside care: A participant-observation study of hospital nurses. *Patient Education Counsel, 48*(2), 107–113.

McCue, H. (1981). Clinical teaching and the nursing process: Implications for nurse teacher education. *Austrian Nurses Journal, 10*(7): 36–37. (PMID: 6908836 [PubMed—indexed for MEDLINE], no abstract available)

Chapter 7
Communication

▼ ▼ ▼ ▼ ▼ ▼ ▼

LEARNING OBJECTIVES

By the end of this chapter, you should be able to:

1. Describe communication development factors.
2. Describe communication structure.
3. Describe communication barriers.
4. Describe therapeutic communication techniques.
5. Implement basic effective communication techniques.
6. Describe effective crisis communication techniques.
7. Describe techniques to improve communication with team members.

KEY TERMS

Action language
Communication
Communication barriers
Intrapersonal communication
Metacommunication
Nonverbal communication
Nurse-client communication
Perception
Social communication
Somatic language
Therapeutic communication
Verbal communication

SCENARIO

Nicole is a new RN who has been paired with a mentor while orienting to a medical floor. Her mentor is trying to do client teaching with a diabetic client that is frequently admitted for the effects of noncompliance with her treatment plan. Nicole notes that her mentor's tone is terse. The mentor's arms are folded across her chest during the exchange. The mentor informs the client's husband that diabetic teaching has been presented to them several times already. The husband looks down at the floor during the exchange.

THINK ABOUT IT

1. What does the term *therapeutic communication* mean to you?
2. In your experience, what type of barriers can occur to prevent effective communication with clients?
3. Identify your own personal communication style. Do your own thoughts and opinions come out in discussions with others? Do you allow others to finish their thoughts before you speak? Do you really listen to what the other person is saying?

INTRODUCTION

Our view of the client determines our communication style.

Clients today are more knowledgeable about disease conditions and health options than they used to be, and they are not as intimidated about entering the health care system as they once were. Even though the nurse-client relationship is an involuntary relationship, clients rely on nurses for guidance, teaching, and assistance to regain or maintain health. Nurses can accomplish these tasks with effective communication skills.

Our view of the client determines our communication style. If we see clients as dependent on us, we may approach them with a one-upmanship manner or, possibly, in a patronizing manner. If we see them as intelligent clients who desire input and partnering in their health care choices, we will communicate with them as equals. We will see ourselves as mentors and guides to assist them with their health issues.

Communication is the essential element in establishing interpersonal relationships and nurse-client relationships. In this chapter we will focus on effectively communicating interpersonally with others—therapeutically with a client, interventionally in a crisis, and competently with other health care team members. We will also briefly discuss developmental factors that affect communication.

$\mathscr{D}$EVELOPMENTAL CONSIDERATIONS

Infants express themselves verbally and nonverbally. They cry when hungry or uncomfortable, thus expressing personal desires with verbal communication. Chitty (1997) describes an infant's nonverbal communication of kicking, turning red in the face, and making facial gestures as **somatic language.**

As the infant progresses into the toddler stage, verbal communication develops by repeating words and then phrases. The toddler also communicates nonverbally with **action language,** such as looking at or pointing to desired objects or holding out a hand for food (Chitty, 1997).

Verbal communication continues to develop as family members verbally stimulate the child. If the child's family is quiet, verbal communication may develop more slowly or inadequately. Nonverbal communication also develops within the environmental setting as the child observes nonverbal communication such as kisses, hugs, and hand gestures (Chitty, 1997). Children take on the observed behaviors and spoken language of their exemplars.

Cultural influences affect communication in words, speed of speech, and gestures. Culture determines distance between individuals during conversation. Some cultures also determine who can speak to whom based on gender or social status.

Communication begins in infancy and is influenced by family and cultural environments. Communication techniques continue to develop from infancy through adulthood. Refer to Table 7–1 for Jean Piaget's

Table 7–1 Piaget's theory of language development

Stage/Age	Piaget's Cognitive Stages
1. Infancy Birth to 1 year	Sensorimotor (birth to 2 years): begins to acquire language Task: Object permanence
2. Toddler 1 to 3 years	Sensorimotor continues Preoperational (2 to 7 years): begins: use of representational thought Task: Use language and mental images to think and communicate
3. Preschool 3 to 6 years	Preoperational continues

4. School Age
6 to 12 years
	Preoperational continues
	Concrete Operations (7 to 12 years)
	    begins: engage in inductive reasoning and concrete
	    problem solving
	Task: Learn concepts of conservation and reversibility

5. Adolescence 12 to 18 years	Formal Operations (12 years to adulthood): engage in abstract reasoning and analytical problem solving Task: Develop a workable philosophy of life

(From *Assessment and Physical Examination* [2nd ed.], by M. Estes, 2002, Albany, NY: Thomson Delmar Learning.)

Theory of Language Development. Effective communication skills are learned depending on desire and practice.

$\mathcal{I}$NTERPERSONAL COMMUNICATION

Communication is the nucleus of relationships and the mechanism by which we influence others.

Communication is the "dynamic interaction between two or more persons in which ideas, goals, beliefs and values, feelings, and feelings about feelings are exchanged" (Hood & Leddy, 2003, p. 453). Communication is the nucleus of relationships and the mechanism by which we influence others. Communication techniques may either develop or fracture personal relationships and nurse-client relationships.

It is vital for nurses to grasp the components of communication and experience the dynamics of effective communication. It is imperative that nurses learn effective communication techniques to develop helping relationships with clients. "The quality of communication between the nurse and the client is an essential determinant of the success of the professional relationship" (Hood & Leddy, 2003, p. 452). Quality relationships with clients determine our influence in assisting the client to a healthier lifestyle.

According to Rowe (1999) the majority of formal complaints at a community health council stemmed from a lack of communication, personnel attitudes, and inappropriate communication of unpleasant news. These communication issues are inappropriate behaviors for caring nurses. Communication consists not only of the spoken word **(verbal communication)** but also of the unspoken word **(nonverbal communication)**. Attitude is communicated in the verbal and the nonverbal message. Attitude also is revealed in the timing, place, and way in which unpleasant news is shared. Caring and communicating are inseparably linked—you cannot hope to communicate effectively if you do not care about the person on the receiving end (Rowe).

CRITICAL THINKING ACTIVITIES

1. Write about a time when a client's attitude hindered the communication process with the health care staff.

_____

_____

_____

2. Write about a time when your attitude affected your communication with a client.

_____

_____

_____

Communication Structure

The sender of a message determines the desired message and encodes the words and gestures with thoughts and feelings. To interpret the message the receiver has to decode the thoughts and feelings in the sender's verbal and nonverbal message.

For communication to occur, there must be a message sender and a message receiver. When we communicate face-to-face, two messages are sent. One is the verbal message of thought and feelings expressed in words influenced by voice volume, inflection, and speech rate. The other message is the nonverbal message or unspoken word expressed with eye movements, gestures, facial expressions, and body movements. Some nonverbal communication needs no spoken word, such as rolling your eyes upward or giving a warm smile.

The sender of a message determines the desired message and encodes the words and gestures with thoughts and feelings. To interpret the message the receiver has to decode the thoughts and feelings in the sender's verbal and nonverbal message. After determining the perceived meaning of the message, the receiver responds to the message by encoding a message with personal thoughts and feelings expressed in words and/or gestures. An interaction occurs between sender and receiver simultaneously. While the sender is sending a message she is interpreting the receiver's message, and as the receiver receives the message she is interpreting and sending a message (Riley, 2000).

To interpret a message, a person analyzes two parts of the message: the message content, and the message's perceived meaning. The message content is what is literally expressed verbally or nonverbally. The message **perception** is how the content is interpreted and how the relationship between the message sender and the message receiver is perceived or emotionally interpreted. To put perceptual meaning to a message is to put meaning to the sensed emotions of the message. Taylor (1997) views perception as something that people learn from their individual socialization experience. Therefore, each person interprets messages according to her learned perceptual ability, causing message interpretation to vary.

Metacommunication

Metacommunication is the message perception of verbal and nonverbal communication. Hood and Leddy (2003) state, "The nurse searches for the content theme (the central underlying idea or links), the mood theme (the emotion communicated—the how of the message), and the interaction theme (the dynamics between the communicating participants)" (p. 457). To communicate effectively, the nurse must comprehend the content of the message, the emotions of the message, and the emotional relationship of the communicators. The nurse must understand the content or key idea that the communicator is attempting to communicate. If the key idea is missed, then communication is misinterpreted by all parties involved. An example of this is the classic Abbott and Costello baseball routine, "Who's on first?"

The nurse needs to be attuned to the manner or emotions in which the message is communicated. For example, she needs to perceive the communicator's anxiety, negativity, excitement, frustration, or fear. The emotions can be displayed by voice fluctuation (voice elevation or a soft, fading voice) and nonverbal communication (looking down, avoiding eye contact, and rolling the eyes).

The emotional relationship of the communicators may depend on past experiences, trust, respect, and cultural practices. If the nurse is attuned to the content of the message, the emotions of the message, and the emotional relationship of the communicators, she will communicate more effectively. Keep in mind that this type of communication will not occur overnight. Communication is a lifelong process and a major component of nursing. Your educational experience in the next few semesters will assist you in identifying the components of communication.

Factors Influencing Message Interpretation

Factors other than the content and emotional aspects of metacommunication can affect communication. Some of these factors influence the sent messages and the interpretation of the messages. Riley (2000) has suggested six factors that influence message interpretation:

1. Environment—temperature, distance between people (across the room or at opposite ends of the table), furniture placement, formal and informal atmosphere.
2. Personal space—rank, position, seating arrangement, physical build (height and weight), touching.
3. Nonverbal—eye movements, gestures, body language, eye contact, crossed arms.
4. Physical appearance—body profile, hair, body movements and gestures, age, gender, posture, body art and piercing.

5. Intrapersonal aspects—speech, values, self-concept, thinking processes, learning styles.

6. "I" messages verses "you" messages.

An example of factors that interfere with message interpretation relating to environment, personal space, and nonverbal communication is a nurse's standing in the doorway with her arms crossed and talking to a client rather than approaching the client's bedside, pulling up a chair, or placing a hand on her arm when talking about the client's concern (Figure 7–1). Most people find the nurse's moving closer to the bed very comforting and conducive to a more positive nurse-client relationship. However, each individual's personal space varies. All health care providers should acknowledge and respect an individual's personal space.

Another situation in which a personal space factor may interfere with message interpretation is a formal atmosphere where a client may hesitate to ask the nurse manager a health-related question due to her position. The client may also hesitate to ask the health question because she does not want to bother the nurse manager or ask her to do something that she does not feel is her responsibility.

Other examples of nonverbal factors are a client's being distracted when a nurse uses excessive hand movements or is overly dramatic when talking. Some clients may become uncomfortable with prolonged eye contact or avoidance of eye contact.

Physical appearance may interfere with message interpretation in a variety of ways. Clients respond very differently to the physical appearance and gender of the nurse. A female client may or may not be open with a male nurse. The nurse's white uniform may comfort some clients and intimidate others.

Intrapersonal aspects are other factors interfering with message interpretation. The self-concept of a nurse or a client can be expressed in a pleasing or intimidating manner that enhances or interferes with communication. It is important to recognize that each individual's learning style varies and affects the way a nurse communicates with a client. A nurse with a concrete learning style might list steps when

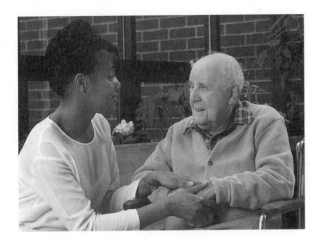

Figure 7–1 Both verbal and nonverbal communication are important in the nurse-client relationship.

explaining a procedure or give more specific directions that seem demanding, whereas a nurse with an abstract learning style might give more descriptive examples when explaining concepts. The nurse with an abstract learning style might take more care with the decorations in a client's room, such as placing cards on a bulletin board or watering the client's flowers.

"I" messages attempt to keep communication open. "You" messages may put a person on the defense. I messages give an individual freedom to express her feelings without blaming others. For example, "I am not sure I see it that way" versus "You are wrong."

It is important that we carefully select the correct words to convey our desired meaning. Messages are often incorrectly interpreted or misunderstood. If we do not understand a message or are not clear as to what is being said or related, we need to validate the meaning of the message with the receiver. Asking "Are you saying . . . ?" or "Do you mean. . . ?" can do this.

The techniques used in interpersonal relationships will assist you as you communicate with clients. Other communication techniques discussed later in the chapter also improve nurse-client relationships.

CRITICAL THINKING ACTIVITY

1. Concentrate on your interactions with others for two days, focusing especially on the content of the message, the emotions of the message, and the emotional relationship of the communicators. Review Riley's six factors that influence communication and determine ways those factors influenced your interactions with others. Complete the following communication chart to analyze two conversations you have with others.

Conversation	Content	Emotions	Emotional relationship	Factors that influenced message interpretation	Perception enhancement/ interference

𝒞OMMUNICATION WITH CLIENTS

Nurse-client communication is the therapeutic inter-action between a nurse and a client that improves the client's physical, emotional, and/or spiritual health.

Nurse-client communication is the therapeutic interaction between a nurse and a client that improves the client's health physically, emotionally, and/or spiritually. Before we discuss effective communication techniques to improve nurse-client communication, let's review some barriers to effective communication.

Communication Barriers

Communication barriers are ineffective phrases or behaviors that damage personal interactions and should be avoided when communicating with clients.

Communication barriers are ineffective phrases or behaviors that damage personal interactions and should be avoided when communicating with clients. Hood and Leddy (2003) refer to these as noncaring communication behaviors. Some of these barriers are responding defensively, blaming, giving advice or opinions, changing the subject, questioning the client, giving judgmental responses, and patronizing (Coordinating Council for Continuing Education in Health Care, 1990).

Blaming statements

Giving advice

Changing the subject or topic

Why questions

Judgmental statements

Patronizing statements

Falsely reassuring statements

Failure to listen

Box 7–1 Barriers to communication

Blaming Statements

Examples of blaming statements are "You made me drop this" or "That is a stupid question you put on this exam. You tried to trick me." No one likes to be blamed for a situation, and a blaming statement places the blame on another person. Blaming statements may cause an individual to respond defensively and in anger. A defensive response is an attempt to protect oneself from a negative opinion. It also denies individuals the right to express their view or opinion of a situation (Hood & Leddy, 2003). It attempts to deflect the statement. Rather than responding defensively with a blaming statement, a person could approach an error, difficult situation, or hurt feelings with an "I" statement or by saying, "How can we handle or repair this situation?"

Giving Advice

If a nurse gives advice or shares her opinion, the client may assume the nurse knows the best option. In essence, the nurse is saying that the client does not have the ability to make wise decisions. An example of giving advice is a scenario in which an elderly client is ready for discharge from the hospital. The physician and family think it is best for the client to be admitted to a nursing home. The client asks the nurse what she thinks. The nurse says, "I think you are capable of caring for yourself at home, especially if you have a home care nurse visit you once a week." The nurse has expressed an opinion and given advice that will confuse the discharge issues.

If a client asks a nurse a question, the nurse's ideal response would be to explore various options with the client and assist the client in making her own decision. In this case, the nurse shows the client she believes that the client is capable of making sound decisions.

Changing the Subject or Topic

A client with cancer says, "I feel like I am getting weaker every day. I wonder if the chemotherapy is working." The nurse responds, "Isn't it beautiful outside today?" This type of nontherapeutic communication is called changing the subject or topic. A nurse may change the topic when the client is sharing personal feelings or thoughts about a subject that make the nurse uncomfortable. When a client is talking and the nurse purposely changes the topic, the client's impression is that the nurse is in charge of discussion topics. Changing the client's topic also negates the importance or value of the client.

Why Questions

A client in a nursing home states, "I don't think you like me." "Now *why* would you think that?" replies the nurse. "Why" statements or questions tend to put the other person on the defensive. The client may think the nurse is probing for more information or questioning her thinking.

Judgmental Statements

When a nurse uses a judgmental statement, she passes judgment on the client or the client's statements. This type of statement judges the client's values and indicates a value difference between nurse and client. The statement implies that the nurse's values, standards, or perceptions are better than the client's. If a client consistently is given judgmental statements, a dependent relationship is fostered because the client begins to think that her opinion has no value and that the other person has all the appropriate knowledge or correct thinking.

Patronizing Statements

A patronizing statement is a demeaning, condescending statement made to another. For example, a nurse may say to a client, "You just don't understand. We always use EKGs in this type of situation." When a nurse uses a patronizing statement, the client receives the impression that the nurse is superior or arrogant and that the nurse and the client are not in an equal position or on an equal playing field. The nurse's communication implies contempt toward the client.

A nurse may fall into the trap of using this type of communication when she has worked in the same place for a long time, has become very knowledgeable, and feels that she knows what is best for the client. If a nurse is in a hurry, she may give a quick, demeaning response instead of giving the client the explanation she is seeking. Instead of assisting the client in understanding, the nurse belittles the client because she does not understand.

Another environment where a nurse might use patronizing communication is communicating with clients who are experiencing changes in mental status, such as someone having an emotional breakdown or in a state of depression. When a client is not thinking as quickly as she used to think or as quickly as we expect her to, the patronizing nurse simply determines the client's needs without involving her in the process. Sometimes as a client ages and becomes more dependent on the health care provider for her activities of daily living, the nurse may assume that her mental capacity has also become reduced, making her more dependent on the nurse. The nurse may cut the client short and give a quick response to what she thinks the client is attempting to say.

Falsely Reassuring Statements

An example of a falsely reassuring statement is, "Oh, everything will be all right. You have the best doctor in town." This negates the client's concerns and fears and makes her hesitant to share other feelings with the nurse. The nurse is failing to assist the client in exploring personal thoughts and feelings. A nurse may use false reassurance when communicating in difficult situations with a grim prognosis, or if she does not recognize the anxiety in a client's statement or question.

Failure to Listen

The most valuable tangible action one individual can give to another is to listen to what that individual is saying.

Failing to listen is the most noncaring communication a nurse can demonstrate (Hood & Leddy, 2003). By failing to listen to the client, the nurse is saying that the client's needs are not important. She may even be implying that her own needs are more important than the client's. This is the behavior of a noncaring nurse. The most valuable tangible action one individual can give to another is to listen to what that individual is saying.

Hood and Leddy (2003) suggest that nurses who use nontherapeutic communication have a need to act in a regressive or retreating manner. "This need, accompanied by increasing anxiety, sometimes leads to nurses seeing themselves as superior, and is expressed in negative actions such as moralizing, rejecting, or reacting with hostility" (pp. 475–476). Learning to communicate therapeutically encourages an individual to look inward as well as learn to listen and respond in a caring, effective way. Communication involves personal analysis, attentive and active listening skills, and meaningful, caring responses.

Therapeutic Communication

Therapeutic communication and social communication are not the same. We use **social communication** in everyday life. Social communication is communication in a less formal environment when we are discussing less personal or serious issues. Social communication is spontaneous and does not have specific goals.

A nurse uses **therapeutic communication** in nurse-client relationships. Therapeutic communication has the client's best interests at heart and is goal oriented. The purpose of therapeutic communication is to enhance and improve communication with clients. Nurses use therapeutic communication when they "carefully [select] communication interventions" (Schuster, 2000, p. 7) to obtain a communication goal. The nurse's therapeutic communication goals are to assist a client to formulate ideas, express those ideas more clearly, and sort through issues to find a solution. Therapeutic communication can also be very effective with other nurses, other health care workers, and even family members.

Nurses demonstrate caring behaviors by avoiding communication barriers and effectively using techniques to improve communication with clients. Some therapeutic communication techniques are broad open-ended statements or questions, reflection, clarification, silence, reassurance, summarization, and acknowledgement (Coordinating Council for Continuing Education in Health Care, 1990).

Broad open-ended statements or questions

Reflection

Clarification

Silence

Reassurance

Summarization

Acknowledgment

Box 7–2 Therapeutic communication techniques

Broad Open-Ended Statements or Questions

A nurse effectively communicates with the client when she uses broad open-ended statements or questions. An example of an open-ended statement is, "Tell me more about . . ." or "Can you explain that to me in another way?" Open-ended statements offer the client an opportunity to guide the direction of the conversation. They allow the client to choose the topic focus and proceed with the conversation. This type of statement shows the client that the nurse is personally interested in her and what she is saying. It also does not put the client on the defensive as a "why," "what," or "how" question does.

Reflection

The nurse uses a reflection statement by restating or rephrasing the client's statement to show interest in the client's concerns and have the client expand on an idea. A client says, "I wish my children would call me. They have been on vacation for two weeks." The nurse would use a reflective statement by saying, "You're missing your children and would like to receive a call from them?" or "You are worried about your children because they're on vacation and you haven't heard from them since they left?" Reflection also allows the nurse to say, "I'm listening. Keep going." This statement reassures the client of the nurse's interest in the client's statements.

Clarification

Clarification is attempting to make the client's meaning clear. With clarification, the nurse usually explains to the client that she desires clarification. The nurse may say, "I want to make sure I understand you correctly. Did you mean . . . ?" Or the nurse could simply say, "You are saying. . . ."

Silence

At times there is no need for verbal communication between client and nurse. The nurse shows client acceptance by silently remaining with the client when she is receiving distressing news (Hood & Leddy, 2003). This way, the nurse is nonverbally indicating a desire to be with the client. Even if she says nothing, the nurse desires to share the moment with the client.

The nurse might use silence when a client receives disappointing news such as a terminal diagnosis or a family death. By remaining at the client's side silently and perhaps holding her hand, the nurse uses silence effectively.

Reassurance

A client has expressed concern about the length of time it is taking to get results from a test. If the nurse were to say, "This is the typical length of time for the test results to be processed," she would be giving the client verbal reassurance. The nurse is not falsely reassuring the client but, rather, giving the client accurate, positive affirmation to ease her concerns.

Summarization

Summarization may be used after a nurse-client teaching session to recap the main points. The nurse may also use summarization after detailed instructions have been given to review the main facts. A nurse's summarization statement could be, "Now I would like to summarize the things we have discussed."

Acknowledgment

> *To be an effective communicator, there must be desire and practice—desire to become an effective communicator, and consistent practice in effectively using the techniques.*

The client feels valued when the nurse acknowledges and addresses her concerns. "I understand you would like to talk with the doctor this morning" is an example of acknowledgment.

To use any of these techniques requires the nurse to listen attentively and actively to the client and to desire to communicate with the client. To be an effective communicator, there must be desire and practice—desire to become an effective communicator, and consistent practice in effectively using the techniques.

CRITICAL THINKING ACTIVITY

1. Write about a professional situation when you experienced any of the following barriers in communicating with a client. Then write how that situation would have been different if you had used any of the following communication techniques.

Barrier to communication	How did the barrier occur?	What was the effect on the communication?
Giving advice		
Changing the subject or topic		
Why questions		
Judgmental statements		
Patronizing statements		
Falsely reassuring statements		
Failure to listen		

Therapeutic communication technique	How did you use the technique?	What was accomplished?
Broad open-ended statements or questions		
Reflection		
Clarification		
Silence		
Reassurance		
Summarization		
Acknowledgment		

CRISIS COMMUNICATION

It is important for the nurse to sense the client's tension and not respond to the situation with personal anxiety.

Hood and Leddy (2003) state, "Anxiety is the tension state resulting from the actual or anticipated negative appraisal of the significant other in the communication process." Anxiety is communicated to the other by voice and nonverbal body language. A client may be anxious if she is anticipating negative news or test results. It is important for the nurse to sense the client's tension and not respond to the situation with personal anxiety. If both parties communicate anxiety, the tension will only escalate.

Anxiety causes the client to ineffectively use energy that is needed to solve a problem or act appropriately (Hood & Leddy, 2003). It is important for both the nurse and the client to channel energy into positive actions. Sullivan (1953) stated that anxiety in limited amounts and duration could lead to increased alertness and energy needed to take appropriate action to reduce tension. If the anxiety is not limited, there may be a decrease in the effectiveness of handling situations. Mild anxiety allows a person to focus on the situation at hand. Moderate anxiety limits an individual's focus and twists reality for her. Severe anxiety does not allow an individual to focus her energy on the real issues and, therefore, limits her problem-solving and decision-making abilities. It is important for the nurse to recognize both her own and the client's anxiety levels to effectively assist in problem solving and decision making. For the client or the nurse to utilize their energy most effectively, anxiety must be decreased. Nurses can learn, use, and share stress-reduction techniques with clients.

Assess a client's anxiety level before starting a teaching session. If the client's anxiety level is moderate to severe, her learning ability will be limited. You can reduce the client's anxiety level with the use of therapeutic communication techniques.

An example of effective therapeutic communication techniques with an anxious client is demonstrated in the scenario in Box 7–3.

Client: "I just don't think I can give myself the insulin injection. I have always been afraid of needles. Even when I was a child, I would become very anxious and scream with injections."

Nurse: "I can see that you are very anxious and it sounds like you have been afraid of needles for a long time. What scares you about the needles?"

Client: "I don't like the pain when I get a shot."

Nurse: "How does the pain from an insulin injection compare to the pain from other injections you have had?"

Client: "I guess the insulin injection really doesn't hurt as bad as the other injections I have had, like antibiotics and pain medication."

Box 7–3 Therapeutic communication scenario

> *Nurse:* "Do you think that if you were in control of the injection, rather than a nurse, you could handle the situation better?"
>
> *Client:* "Now, I hadn't thought of that idea. I actually can be in control of the insulin injection."
>
> *Nurse:* (after a slight pause) "Do you feel comfortable trying the injection now?"

Box 7–3 (continued)

COMMUNICATING AS A TEAM MEMBER

A judicious nurse does not drop the effective communication skills at the client's bedside but continues to apply them in interacting with health care team members (Chitty, 1997).

We have discussed interpersonal communication techniques, therapeutic communication techniques, and nontherapeutic communication techniques. Nurses must communicate effectively not only with clients but also with members of the health care team. Many of the same techniques we use in interpersonal communication and therapeutic communication can be used with team members. A judicious nurse does not drop the effective communication skills at the client's bedside but continues to apply them in interacting with health care team members (Chitty, 1997).

Some communication enhancement techniques the nurse could use with team members are active listening, respect of others, spacing and distance, attention to nonverbal communication cues, "I" messages, and avoidance of communication "barriers." The nurse is not attempting to accomplish the same goals of therapeutic communication with team members that are accomplished in nurse-client interactions. However, effective communication techniques used with clients can be carried over into conversation with team members. Communicating in concise, well thought-out, simple messages can enhance communication personally and professionally.

Trust and support are vital for a smooth, efficient working environment. Effective communication can provide these encouraging factors. As team members sense trust and support, they will feel free to share creative ideas and suggestions for change. In an accepting environment, employees will gain job satisfaction and they will blossom.

The nursing shortage and early hospital discharges have added more stress to the clinical environment. Effective communication skills such as clarification, reflection, and reassurance decrease tension in stressful situations.

Self-Talk

How a person feels about self determines the portrayal of self to others in appearance, body carriage, gestures, and expression.

Self-assessment, self-worth, and self-talk can have a definite effect on team member communication. Kearney (2001) calls the "way one communicates with self, or self-talk" **intrapersonal communication** (p. 148). How a person feels about self determines the portrayal of self to others in appearance, body carriage, gestures, and expression. If a nurse has a negative encounter with a manager, the nurse's thoughts and talk may tend to take on a negative air. It is important at that point to assess personal accountability for the encounter candidly and make amends as needed. Self-talk is also important to instill positive input back into self. The self-talk will influence future interactions with other team members that could be negatively or positively influenced by the self-talk (Kearney).

Body Language

Ineffective body language that affects communication is crossing the arms, indicating rejection or closed-mindedness; biting fingernails, signifying nervousness; and turning the body away from the other person, representing boredom, rejection, or conflict. Portraying a relaxed attitude and demeanor is generally positive (Kearney, 2001). It is also important to be genuine.

CRITICAL THINKING ACTIVITY

1. Relate two interactions with a team member when you and/or other team members implemented at least two communication techniques. How did the communication techniques hinder or improve the communication?

First interaction	Communication technique implemented	Communication technique's effect on the interaction
Second interaction	Communication technique implemented	Communication technique's effect on the interaction

$\mathscr{S}$UMMARY

Communication dramatically affects personal and professional relationships. Communication is not only the words you speak, but also how you express those words verbally and nonverbally. As nurses, our communication skills will be important in everything we do. Our professional role often elicits an automatic respect or trust from clients. We must be responsible in that role and always strive to communicate in a therapeutic manner. It is important for us to evaluate how we communicate with others, to change what is not effective, and to develop and implement effective communication techniques.

$\mathscr{C}$HAPTER REFLECTIONS

1. What is the mentor's nonverbal communication saying in the chapter scenario?
2. Is therapeutic conversation occurring between the mentor and the client's husband?

3. What are some of the barriers to therapeutic communication in the scenario?

4. Do you think that this communication interaction with the client and her husband will promote compliance? Why or why not?

REFERENCES

Chitty, K. (1997). *Professional nursing: concepts and challenges* (2nd ed.). Philadelphia: W.B. Saunders Company.

Coordinating Council for Continuing Education in Health Care. (1990). *Barriers and bridges on the road to better communication* [Motion picture]. University Park, PA: Pennsylvania State University.

Hood, L., & Leddy, S. (2003). *Leddy and Pepper's conceptual bases of professional nursing* (5th ed.). Philadelphia: Lippincott Williams & Wilkins.

Kearney, R. (2001). *Advancing your career: Concepts of professional nursing.* Philadelphia: F.A. Davis Company.

Riley, J. (2000). *Communication in nursing* (4th ed.). St. Louis, MO: Mosby.

Rowe, J. (1999, November 10–16). Self-awareness: Improving nurse-client interactions. *Nursing Standard* [On-line]. Available: http://80-proquest.umi .com

Schuster, P. (2000). *Communication: The key to the therapeutic relationship.* Philadelphia: F.A. Davis.

Sullivan, H. (1953). *The interpersonal theory of psychiatry.* New York: Norton.

Taylor, A. (1997). *Communicating.* Englewood Cliffs, NJ: Prentice Hall.

SUGGESTED RESOURCES

Breisch, L. (1999). Motivate! *Nursing Management, 30*(3), 27–30.

Chant, S. (2002). Communication skills: Some problems in nursing education and practice. *Journal of Clinical Nursing, 11*(1), 12–21 [On-line]. Available: http://lore.inspire.net

Communicating and managerial effectiveness. (2003). *Nursing Management, 9*(9), 30–35.

Costello, M. (2001). Improving communications key for workforce. *AHA News 37*(27), 5.

Dreachslin, J., Hunt, P., & Sprainer, E. (1999). Key indicators of nursing care team performance: Insights from the front line. *The Health Care Supervisor 12*(4), 70–76.

Meadows, G., & Chaiken, B. (2003). Using IT to improve clinical teamwork and communication. *Nursing Economics, 21*(1), 33–35.

Peterson, L., Halsey, J., Albrecht, T., & McGough, K. (1995). Communicating with staff nurses: Support or hostility? *Nursing Management, 26*(6), 36–38.

$\mathscr{P}$ART III
The Nurse as Manager

▼ ▼ ▼ ▼ ▼ ▼ ▼

*C*hapter 8
The Nurse as Leader

▼ ▼ ▼ ▼ ▼ ▼ ▼

*L*EARNING OBJECTIVES

By the end of this chapter, you should be able to:

1. Define leadership.
2. Define manager.
3. Explain different leadership theories.
4. Explain different leadership styles.
5. Explain different management theories.
6. Define basic concepts of nurses in leadership roles.
7. Define the differences between LPN and RN leadership roles and responsibilities.

*K*EY TERMS

Accountability

Delegation

Facilitation

Interdependence

Leader

Leadership style

Manager

Mutuality

*S*CENARIO

Tony is not looking forward to the charge role as a new RN. He has always hated "telling people what to do." He would prefer to just take care of his clients. He is wondering how one attains the ability to be in charge. He feels he does not have the qualities to be in charge because he has never been an assertive person. The one time Tony had to be in charge as an LPN, he had a hard time making assignments and assigning tasks. He cannot picture himself in the charge role. He is wondering what else is involved with being a manager. His classmate, Chance, cannot wait to be in charge. He feels it is his turn to get to tell people what to do. These are two very different views. Just what does being a leader mean? What qualities does it take to be a successful manager? Is it more than just telling people what to do?

*T*HINK ABOUT IT

1. Do you think being a leader means telling people what to do?
2. Do you feel that Tony or Chance has an appropriate perception of a leader role?
3. What qualities do you appreciate in a nurse leader?

*I*NTRODUCTION

Growth into leadership can be compared to a flower's petals continually opening in slow motion. As each petal unfolds, the leader gains knowledge, matures, expands, takes risks, is challenged in new ways, and constantly goes for the goal. Just as most flower petals do not go back into a tight bud, so the leader cannot take back his mistakes or blunders but must continue to unfold and find new ways to handle the unremitting challenges of the job. The bud may develop into a beautiful bloom, and the leader into an effective facilitator. Sometimes frost or insects make dark spots on some of the petals. Rough times in leadership make dark spots in the leader's mind and heart and scar them. Yet the petals continue to unfold, and the leader grows, and the job presents more challenges.

The role of the leader has blossomed, changed, and evolved over the years, and the complex concept of leadership is still evolving and conforming to societal changes. Gregory-Dawes stated in "Changing Times, Changing Roles" (2000) that because of business influences on health care, "Managerial responsibilities were expected to change from that of sole decision makers to supportive, coaching, and nurturing roles" (p. 177).

In this chapter we will define leadership and management and explore the role of the RN as leader and manager. We will discuss the role of delegation and define accountability as they relate to leadership and management. We will also review the impact of the nursing shortage on nursing leadership and nursing in general. We will explain different leadership styles and briefly discuss some leadership and management theories.

ℒEADERSHIP THEORIES

Leadership theories generally reflect the changing attitudes of each generation toward leadership styles and behaviors.

Leadership styles and behaviors have been studied for years, and several theories have developed over time. Leadership theories generally reflect the changing attitudes of each generation toward leadership styles and behaviors. Some leadership theories are 1) the traditional views of leadership, 2) transformational leadership theory, 3) leadership tasks theory, and 4) new science leadership theory.

Traditional Views of Leadership

The traditional concept of a leader was one who had a vision or knew a direction to take and interacted with and motivated others to reach the goal.

Asselin (2001) described a leader as one who "sets the vision, tone, and direction" (p. 24). Epstein (1982) defined leadership as a process of "influencing individuals or groups to take an active part in the process of achieving agreed-upon goals" (p. 2). The traditional concept of a leader was one who had a vision or knew a direction to take and interacted with and motivated others or the followers to reach the vision or goal.

For a leader to lead there must be followers. The relationship between leader and followers is crucial to the success of the leader. The leader has a plan and a goal, but the relationship with the followers determines whether the leader reaches that goal. The followers must desire to follow the leader, and the leader must motivate and guide the followers.

Transformational Leadership Theory

The transformational leadership theory defines the leader as drawing strength from personal values, having a vision, and interacting with collaborators.

Rost (1994) saw the term *follower* as describing a "submissive and inactive" role and continued to define leadership as "an influence relationship among leaders and collaborators who intend real changes that reflect their mutual purposes"(p. 3). This more current definition of leadership involves empowerment and mutual goal setting and is known as transformational leadership. Rost's definition uses the term *collaborators* rather than *followers,* indicating mutuality in goal setting and goal attainment. Kearney (2001) states that "the transformational leader operates out of a deeply held personal value system, is visionary, has strong convictions, and interacts significantly with followers to see that the vision is realized" (p. 229). To refine this definition for more current concepts, we would define the leader as drawing strength from personal values, having a vision, and interacting with collaborators. Personal beliefs and values and past experiences set the tone for the leader's leadership style.

It is vital for the transformational leader to take the pulse of all collaborators consistently. Are all individuals willing to be a part of the team? Do some of the individuals have different goals than stated or than others in the group? Do some individuals have their own agenda? A leader needs to listen attentively to the verbal and nonverbal communication of the team members. When listening, the leader needs to clarify what is being said to fully comprehend the message being sent. It is important to assess the team frequently.

Leadership Tasks Theory

John Gardner, the developer of the leadership tasks theory, listed nine tasks of a leader (1990). These leadership tasks are envisioning goals, affirming values, motivating, managing, achieving workable unity, explaining and teaching, serving as a symbol, representing the group, and renewing (Gardner, n.d.).

The first task, envisioning goals, involves setting goals and motivating others to achieve those goals. This is the heart and soul of a leader. The leader must know what he wants to accomplish and how to get there. The goal must be so clear that he can communicate it to others and inspire them to achieve the goal. Some leaders have vision that extends beyond their time and can influence many generations. Florence Nightingale is an example of such a leader:

> One of the purest examples of the leader as agenda setter was Florence Nightingale. Her public image was and is that of the lady of mercy, but under her gentle manner, she was a rugged spirit, a fighter, a tough-minded system changer. She never made public appearances or speeches, and except for her two years in the Crimea, held no public position. Her strength was that she was a formidable authority on the evils to be remedied, she knew what to do about them, and she used public opinion to goad top officials to adopt her agenda. (Gardner, 1990, pp. 15–16)

Every community has beliefs, ideas, and customs it holds dear. A leader sanctions and believes in the values and norms of the community. In the leadership role, the leader represents and affirms the community's values in the people.

According to the leadership tasks theory the leader does not force the people to action but motivates them to action.

Gardner (1990) states that leaders "unlock or channel existing motives" (p. 14). Leaders are able to harness the desires and will of people and make them move toward the established goals of the leader or group. Ideally, the leader does not force people to action but motivates them to action.

Managing includes five steps for the leader: planning and priority setting, organizing and institution building, keeping the system functioning, agenda setting and decision making, and exercising political judgment. Once the leader has set the goals, someone must plan the steps, set the path, and shift priorities to accomplish the goals. A leader does not center the focus on himself but establishes the goals, motivates, and instills direction in others, thus building an "institution" of the people. Then if something happens to the leader the institution carries on the action. During the Great Depression, President Franklin Roosevelt encouraged, inspired, and motivated the American people to press on for success. After his death, many future generations were influenced by his vision. To keep the system functioning, the leader provides resources, supplies staff, directs, guides, develops procedures, delegates, coordinates, and keeps the system productive. Some leaders have a goal and can visualize the fulfillment of the goal, but they may lack the ability to plan the step-by-step process to reach the goal. The leader who is not a detailed person will need to draft others to assist him in determining the step-by-step activities to achieve the goal. The leader exercises political judgment by preventing conflicts from interfering with the accomplishment of the goal.

The leader strives to achieve a workable unity. Conflict does not have to be viewed as a negative but can be seen as a stimulant or a challenge. The leader determines whether an issue is a conflict or a lack of cooperation from the group. Part of the leader's time is spent in establishing and maintaining unity in the group.

Great leaders are willing to explain, explain, and reexplain. People want to know the rationale behind their being asked to do certain things, and why things are being done in a specific manner. Clear, candid, concise explanations will assist the leader in developing unity. The people want and need to be kept informed.

The leader represents the members of the group both within the group and outside of the group. What he does and says represents the group. The leader does not represent his personal desires or thoughts but speaks and thinks as the group when he acts on its behalf in an outside context.

The leader needs to have a global focus. Sometimes a leader can lead the people down a tried and true, unchanging path. However, he must constantly be aware of the new thoughts and technology that are available and keep abreast of new and better ways to accomplish new goals.

According to leadership tasks theory, a leader does not have to be in an appointed position to lead others. Nurses can apply this theory to their own lives by remembering that they do not have to be appointed to a leadership position to lead. By applying any of these principles, they are acting as leaders and can make the nursing profession better and improve client care.

New Science Leadership Theory

> *The new science leadership theory emphasizes that the leader must value and establish relationships with an acceptance of the values of all members.*

The concepts of the new science leadership theory are coherent with the transformational leadership theory and leadership tasks theory. Wheatley (1992) presented the new science leadership theory, emphasizing that the leader must value and establish relationships with an acceptance of the values of all members. He also viewed chaos as productive and inevitable in an ever-changing, evolving world. An environment where members are valued produces flexibility and an openness to change. It also encourages the exchange of ideas and creativity. This leadership style is the essence of collaboration. Brandt, Holt, and Sullivan, in "How to Make Conflict Work for You" (2001), state, "Where collaboration reigns, strife wanes" (p. 32). A collaborative leadership style takes longer to develop and achieve but fosters individual growth, empowerment, and self-esteem.

CRITICAL THINKING ACTIVITIES

1. Write your definition of a leader.

   _____

   _____

   _____

2. Review your personal definition of a leader. Which leadership theory does it best fit?

   _____

   _____

   _____

3. In your opinion, which leadership theory has the best fit with the nursing profession?

   _____

   _____

   _____

4. We said above that "conflict does not have to be viewed as a negative but can be seen as a stimulant or a challenge." Think

of a conflict in your life. How could this conflict situation be approached as a stimulant or challenge? If the conflict is viewed as a stimulant or challenge, how will that change you?

_____

_____

_____

5. Do you agree with Brandt, Holt, and Sullivan's statement, "Where collaboration reigns, strife wanes?" Give the rationale for your answer.

_____

_____

_____

ℒEADERSHIP STYLES

Leadership style is the way an individual fulfills his responsibilities regarding the fulfillment of needs, distribution of power, decision-making ability of the group, and attainment of goals.

Leadership is a learned process. Leadership can be learned from examples of previous leaders, examples within the home or social environment, or textbook discussions of leadership. **Leadership style** is the way an individual fulfills his responsibilities regarding the fulfillment of needs, distribution of power, decision-making ability of the group, and attainment of goals. A person's leadership style evolves from personal values, past experiences, and previous work environments. These previous influences form one's concept of the way a leader should lead.

There are three basic leadership styles: _autocratic, laissez-faire,_ and _democratic._ The autocratic or authoritarian leader dominates, controls, gives orders, and expects the orders to be followed. There is little doubt as to who is in charge. The leader is task oriented. Decisions are made from the top downward, generally without consulting the workers. The needs of individual group members are not considered. Often this type of leader lacks effective communication skills. When referring to the work environment, the words he most frequently uses are _I, my,_ and _mine._ The autocratic leader has difficulty adapting to new concepts, ideas, or options. Autocratic leadership style squelches creativity and makes workers feel stymied and controlled. It diminishes individual initiative.

The laissez-faire style of leadership is at the opposite end of the continuum from the autocratic leadership style. In this style of leadership, it is difficult to identify the leader because he is passive and provides little direction to the group. The leader relies on the strengths of each individual to meet loosely defined goals. The group has total autonomy and may lack direction. Laissez-faire leadership may work if the individuals have worked together for a long period of time, know the group goals, and are well motivated. Otherwise, individuals may become complacent and dissatisfied.

The democratic style of leadership is also known as the *collaborative* or *participative* style. The democratic leader makes the final decision after gathering the input and ideas of the group. The leader recognizes that the staff often has the best ideas to attain the goals. More time is consumed in obtaining each individual's ideas, but each person can buy in to the project or goal and feels that he is a part of the team. The words most often used by this leader are *we* and *our*. If there is conflict in the group, the democratic approach may not be the most effective style of leadership. It takes time to create a collaborative, trusting atmosphere in which the staff trusts the leader. This democratic, collaborative environment encourages others within the group to develop their leadership abilities. Group and individual efforts are generously acknowledged and applauded. The leader is an effective communicator and has the healthy self-esteem necessary to admit and own errors as they occur.

Sometimes leaders use different leadership styles in varied circumstances. For instance, in critical situations an authoritarian approach may be more appropriate. In noncritical situations, a democratic approach may be more appropriate.

One philosophy of nursing leadership is explained in the following quotation:

> The "command and control" style that has been a strong component of the leadership/management culture of nursing for much of our history just doesn't work anymore. Leadership is effective only if it can create a positive, supportive environment that frees people to do their best creative work. No longer do we believe that all of the knowledge of how things should be done is invested solely in the leader or manager. (Kerfoot, 1998, p. 180)

Successful leaders utilize the talents and skills of those they lead. Table 8–1 recaps the three basic leadership styles.

Table 8–1 Comparison of leadership styles

	Fulfillment of needs	Distribution of power	Decision-making ability of the group	Attainment of goals	Communication skills	Flexibility
Autocratic	Group member needs are not considered. Individual initiative is diminished. Creativity is squelched.	Leader gives orders.	Decisions are made from top downward without consulting the group.	Leader is task oriented.	Most frequently used words are *I, my,* and *mine.* Leader is often a poor, ineffective communicator.	Creativity is squelched. Leader has difficulty adapting to new concepts, ideas, or options.
Democratic	Group and individual efforts are generously acknowledged and applauded. Leader admits and owns errors as they occur.	Encourages others within the group to develop their leadership abilities. Each person buys in to the project and goal and feels part of the team. Staff trusts the leader.	Leader makes final decision after gathering the input and ideas of the group.	Leader recognizes that staff often has the best ideas.	Most frequently used words are *we* and *our.* Leader is an effective communicator.	Time is taken to obtain each individual's ideas.

| Laissez-faire | Individuals may become complacent and dissatisfied. | Difficult to determine the leader
Leader is passive and provides little direction to the group. | Leader relies on the strengths of each individual to meet loosely defined goals.
Group has total autonomy and may lack direction. | Attained only if group knows goals and are well motivated | Group oriented | Extremely flexible
Produces the most individual creativity. |

CRITICAL THINKING ACTIVITIES

1. We defined leadership style as the way an individual fulfills his responsibilities regarding the fulfillment of needs, distribution of power, decision-making ability of the group, and attainment of goals. Do you agree or disagree with this definition? What would you change in the definition? What would you add to the definition? Discuss the leadership style definition with your peers.

   _____

   _____

   _____

2. What leadership style do you prefer? Discuss your rationale. What life influences have led to your preference?

   _____

   _____

   _____

3. In your opinion, do the business and technology professions need a different type of leadership style than the nursing profession? Give the rationale for your answer.

   _____

   _____

   _____

MANAGEMENT THEORIES

We will briefly discuss two management theories: *scientific management* and *human relations–oriented management*. The scientific management theory is task oriented. A scientific manager would focus on the results: number of clients provided with care, number of procedures each nurse performs, adequate equipment to do the job, and documentation of work accomplished by each staff member.

The human relations–oriented manager would be concerned about employee morale and would make every effort to keep employees motivated to do their best. This type of manager cares about employees' hopes, dreams, and concerns. He makes every effort to work out conflict in a smooth and efficient manner. If employees are content, the manager believes they will do their best work. The human relations–oriented manager cares about quality client care and an efficiently running unit but believes that contented employees make the unit more efficient and productive.

CRITICAL THINKING ACTIVITIES

1. Write your own definition of a manager.

   _____

   _____

   _____

2. Review your definition of a manager. Which management theory does it best fit?

   _____

   _____

   _____

3. In your opinion, which management theory is best suited for the nursing profession? Give the rationale for your answer.

   _____

   _____

   _____

*D*IFFERENCES BETWEEN LEADERSHIP AND MANAGEMENT

A leader seeks input from and collaborates with all members of the team, guiding them toward mutually agreed-upon goals. A manager values individuals' needs while planning the tasks to accomplish the team's goals.

A **leader** seeks input from and collaborates with all members of the team, guiding them toward mutually agreed-upon goals. A **manager** values individuals' needs while planning the tasks to accomplish the team's goals. The leader is a facilitator and a guide. The leader does not disdain chaos as an enemy but sees it as an opportunity to grow, change, and remain flexible to meet the needs of the ever-changing environment. The manager component of leadership is more task or planning oriented than the leader component but must not eliminate the value and needs of the team members in accomplishing the plan.

$\mathscr{T}$HE RN AS LEADER

Leadership concepts include empowerment, advocacy, mutuality, facilitation, professionalism, communication, teaching, interdependence, resource development and management, delegation, and accountability.

According to Morgan (2000), "approximately one third of all nurses in management positions in the United States have associate degrees as their highest nursing-related educational preparation" (p. 181). Generally, management prefers that nurses in leadership have at least a baccalaureate degree and encourages nurses in leadership positions to attain higher degrees.

In the past, the leader or manager generally had a title to accompany the position. The business and technology concepts of cost containment, quality outcomes, and customer service have entered the health care arena. With these business and technology influences and the nursing shortage, health care management has had to revamp unit staffing and the utilization of equipment and supplies. According to Gregory-Dawes (2000), "Leaders without titles surfaced and showed their abilities to improve outcomes" (p. 177). In the health care setting, staff nurses started taking on leadership roles, and management was open to these changes in an attempt to cut costs as it provided quality client care.

Leadership concepts include empowerment, advocacy, mutuality, facilitation, professionalism, communication, teaching, interdependence, resource development and management, delegation, and accountability. These leadership concepts will become reality as you take on these leadership roles as an associate degree RN.

Empowerment

In current leadership trends, power is shared. Staff nurses share leadership roles. At some hospitals, one staff nurse may be in charge of a unit one day, and the next day another nurse may share that responsibility. In this way, leaders are developed and nurses who have leadership abilities have an opportunity to exercise their leadership skills.

Knowledge is power. Nurse leaders continually seek out opportunities to increase their knowledge base. Not only do they accumulate knowledge, but they also share this knowledge with other nurses and clients and empower them.

Nurses empower clients by guiding them to discuss their condition openly with the physician. Often, clients are hesitant to approach their physician or discuss treatment plans. The nurse can explain the disease process so that the client has a knowledge-based understanding of his condition and then guide the client in appropriate discussion and treatment approaches with the physician. As your knowledge increases regarding disease pathophysiology and treatment options, you will be able to instruct your clients more thoroughly in their disease conditions.

Advocacy

Nurses spend quality time with clients, and often during this time clients share their treatment desires and wishes. The nurse can become an advocate for the client by relating these desires to the physician or facilitating opportunities for the client to communicate his desires to the physician.

A nurse is an advocate for those who do not have access to care. A nurse advocate takes action when clients are shortchanged because of policies whose taproots are embedded in cost containment.

As LPNs, many of you have functioned as advocates. In most of these situations you accomplished the advocate role by reporting to and collaborating with an RN or other members of the health care team. As you become an RN, you will be responsible in and oversee situations in which you or others will be the client advocate.

Mutuality

Mutuality is the joint sharing of power, resources, and knowledge. Staff nurses must have mutual trust in one another for this to work well. As the leaders on the unit promote and exhibit mutuality, other staff will grow into this camaraderie style of leadership. As an RN, you will have the resources and knowledge to become a leader who promotes mutuality.

Mutuality also extends from nurse to client. With the development of technology, clients are much more knowledgeable about their disease conditions than they were in the past. Therefore there is a mutual sharing of knowledge and acceptance between nurse and client. In mutuality, nurses see the client as having the control and ability to manage the treatment regimen. The client views the nurse as a facilitator in the treatment process. The nurse seeks increased knowledge about the disease process, searches for resources to meet the client needs, and assists the client to gain maximum outcomes.

Facilitation

The nurse acts as a facilitator not only for the client but also for colleagues. **Facilitation** means to assist, ease the way, or make a smooth transition for a process or another person. The associate degree nurse orients new employees to the unit. He eases the transition to the new working environment by teaching the philosophy of the unit, acting as a role model, and orienting the new nurse to the routines of the floor.

The associate degree nurse facilitates the workload of other nurses. He makes suggestions to improve client care, decrease workloads, and make more appropriate use of resources. The goal is to make the unit run smoothly and efficiently for both nurses and clients.

Professionalism

The RN has more autonomy than the LPN in decision making and is accountable for the decisions made.

The nurse leader draws from an underlying knowledge of personal values and needs. He knows why he went into nursing and what drives him to return to work each day. He knows the value of the client and desires to deliver quality care. When times get rough, he reviews why he chose nursing as a profession. When the morale on the unit starts to sag, he reminds other nurses of the opportunities of the nursing profession and stimulates them to do their best.

The LPN is part of the nursing team and is a professional. Generally, the LPN's role is defined as task oriented, meaning that the LPN concentrates on completing assigned nursing tasks. The RN's professional role includes decision making and problem solving. The LPN makes basic decisions and reports and collaborates with the RN in making more detailed decisions. The RN has more autonomy than the LPN in decision making and is accountable for the decisions made. Because of the RN's responsibility for decision making, it is vital that he continually update his knowledge base. The professional RN applies research to practice and keeps abreast of new issues in the nursing profession.

Communication

The associate degree education prepares the LPN for a more effective communication style. Therapeutic communication is listening and effectively smoothing the way for a client to express verbal and non-verbal feelings and thoughts. It involves trust, empathy, listening, and respect. This style of communication encourages the nurse to truly listen to the client, offer every opportunity for the client to verbalize concerns, and clarify communication between nurse and client. Therapeutic communication takes practice and effort and constantly needs refining. Hopefully, the nurse will become so comfortable with therapeutic communication techniques that he will incorporate them into everyday life and utilize them with co-workers, family members, and friends. Nurses can eliminate much conflict by listening and clarifying communication with co-workers.

Gossip has no place in the conversation of the nurse leader. The leader avoids discussing co-workers with other nurses at all costs. Gossip is one vice that can quickly break cohesiveness on the unit. Good communicators can avoid gossip by clarifying meanings with others or speaking candidly *to* the appropriate person rather than *about* the person.

Teaching

Leading is teaching.

Leading is teaching. Nursing leaders teach graduates, new staff, and clients. For nurses, many co-worker and client interactions throughout the day are teaching opportunities. Teaching is explaining information to all involved parties. It is important for a leader to explain to co-workers the rationale behind decisions, schedules, and assignments. The staff wants and needs communication from its leaders. Kerfoot (1998) states that "teaching is the central activity of winning organizations" (p. 181).

As you transition into the RN role, you will become a leader and be responsible for teaching clients, clients' families, and colleagues. As an RN, you may be in charge of a unit, where teaching takes on an even bigger role.

Interdependence

Interdependence is reliance, mutual sharing, mutual assistance, and confidence that the other person will provide support when needed. No one nurse can care for all the clients and make the unit run smoothly. Nurse leaders recognize and promote co-worker interdependence. Kerfoot (1998) states, "Creativity does not exist in hostile environments where all of one's time is spent thinking about survival. The design of nonhierarchical organizations can lead to workplaces where relationships are easy to develop and interdependence rather than independence is the norm" (p. 181). Interdependence promotes a creative, cohesive work environment.

During the LPN-RN educational experience, you probably will work in groups on projects or reports. These group interactions will prepare you for the interdependent role of an RN leader.

Resource Development and Management

As a leader it is important to manage client care resources conscientiously.

According to Kerfoot, "Leaders bring information in and must also send people out to get more [information]" (1998, p. 181). Information is an important resource. Only as leaders continually seek new information and begin utilizing the information can organizations be on the cutting edge of development. A leader shares potential opportunities and encourages participation in continuing education activities. It is important for leaders and staff nurses to participate regularly in seminars and conferences and to keep up to date with the current literature.

As a leader it is important to manage client care resources conscientiously. Nurses need to watch for ways to decrease costs to the client and for the facility. These measures should not decrease the quality of care or jeopardize client outcomes. As an LPN you were aware of costs to clients, but as you assume the RN role you are becoming responsible for finding the most cost-effective ways to provide continuing education for all staff members and quality client care.

Delegation

The nurse leader is knowledgeable about the nurse practice act and the scope of practice for those to whom he is delegating.

Delegation is assigning responsibilities to competent and qualified individuals for satisfactory completion. It is impossible for one person to accomplish all the daily tasks without the assistance of the health care team. Therefore, it is vital to learn the skill and diplomacy of delegation. Not only do nurse leaders delegate, but delegation also takes place at all levels of the health care team. As you transition from LPN to RN, your ability to delegate will become even more valuable to your success as a nurse leader.

The nurse leader is knowledgeable about the nurse practice act and the scope of practice for those to whom he is delegating. Prior to delegating, he considers the strengths and weaknesses of each individual. He does not hesitate to delegate responsibilities to qualified employees within their scope of practice. The nurse leader is legally responsible for the outcomes of the delegated tasks. He distributes work assignments to all employees fairly and treats all employees with respect. The leader does not delegate jobs that he himself would not be willing to perform. He communicates his expectations for the job so that the job is completed appropriately. The nurse leader makes sure the employee has the needed resources to complete the job adequately. He trusts that the employee will do his best in completing the task and relies on him to complete it. Together, the leader and the employee review the outcomes of the delegated work. The leader gladly recognizes and celebrates the employee's accomplishments.

Accountability

The RN's ability to communicate and make wise decisions will be vital as he becomes accountable for the decision made and communicated.

The terms *responsibility* and *accountability* are often used interchangeably because they have similar meanings. Responsibilities are the actual tasks that have been assigned. **Accountability** is being responsible and liable for one's personal actions and for the inaction of oneself and those under supervision. A person can delegate a task but cannot delegate accountability for task completion.

The nurse is accountable for the consequences of all his actions. He provides the best care to the assigned client that he is capable of providing and is held accountable for that care. Accountability to clients includes providing ample care to clients to meet their needs. It also includes obtaining resources to meet the client's needs that the nurse is unable to meet, such as physical therapy, diabetic teaching, or social services. Nurses are responsible for educating the community so that lay people can make appropriate health decisions. Educating the community provides individuals with an opportunity to have a healthier lifestyle and decreased health care costs.

Nurses have a responsibility to participate in political efforts to assure adequate health care to everyone. This could include educating the community on political issues that will affect their health and health care. The nurse functions as the client advocate in political situations and direct nursing care. Nurses are accountable for the quality of health care provided.

Accountability involves practicing safely within the job description of the agency according to the Nurse Practice Act and the nurses' scope of practice. If the job description is inappropriate, measures should be taken to correct its inadequacies. Accountability includes giving an employer an adequate quantity and quality of completed work.

The nurse is accountable not only to the nursing profession but also to himself and his family. It is important to frequently assess whether the personal wellness needs of self and family are being met.

LPNs are accountable for the quality of care provided clients. In transitioning into the RN role, the LPN's accountability will increase. The RN is accountable for larger numbers of clients and for the staff providing care to the clients. The RN's ability to communicate and make wise decisions will be vital as he becomes accountable for the decision made and communicated.

CRITICAL THINKING ACTIVITY

1. Give an example of an RN you have observed exercising each of these leadership concepts. State how each concept is exercised differently by an RN as opposed to an LPN.

   • Empowerment:

   _____

   _____

   _____

   • Advocacy:

   _____

   _____

   _____

   • Mutuality:

   _____

   _____

   _____

   • Facilitation:

   _____

   _____

   _____

   • Professionalism:

   _____

   _____

   _____

   • Communication:

   _____

   _____

   _____

- Teaching:

_____

_____

_____

- Interdependence:

_____

_____

_____

- Resource development and management:

_____

_____

_____

- Delegation:

_____

_____

_____

- Accountability:

_____

_____

_____

*T*HE RN AS MANAGER

Traditional management theories focused on tasks. The contemporary view is that a manager focuses on planning, monitoring results, decision making, decision analysis, resource control, and development.

Traditional management theories focused on tasks. The contemporary view is that a manager focuses on planning, monitoring results, decision making, decision analysis, resource control, and development. Kearney states that "a manager focuses on directing the group to meet the desired outcomes for the organization through thoughtful and careful planning, direction, monitoring, recognition, development, and representation" (2001, p. 257). This definition includes the human relationship component of a manager.

Some literature implies that the manager is an appointed position. Here, we take the approach that an RN can be in an appointed position but that staff nurses also have managerial skills. To be a successful manager one must be results oriented; however, to be only task or results oriented negates the human interaction needed for a collaborative working environment.

Mintzberg (1975) states that there are four managerial roles: *interpersonal, informational, decisional,* and *entrepreneurial.* The interpersonal role deals with developing productive relationships, conflict management, and employee growth. The informational role involves being a representative for staff and administration, relaying information appropriately, and monitoring the progress of the staff and unit. In the decisional role, the manager evaluates employees, monitors budget issues, and resolves conflicts. In the entrepreneurial role, the manager keeps abreast of new concepts and ideas to make the unit effective and profitable.

$\mathscr{S}$UMMARY

Nursing will present the RN leader with many challenges and constant change.

As you transition from your current LPN role into the new role of associate degree RN, it is very important to take time to review the qualities and responsibilities of a mature nurse leader. Nursing will present the RN leader with many challenges and constant change. Through these challenges and changes, the RN will choose the appropriate leadership style and learn the best way to facilitate and guide, collaborate, and communicate with the health care team in order to provide the best possible care to each individual. Model nurse leaders have gleaned knowledge from their surroundings and bloomed into respected and admirable leaders who make a difference in the nursing world.

$\mathscr{C}$HAPTER REFLECTIONS

1. How have your perceptions of the leader role changed?
2. What positive qualities can you identify in yourself that will help you to assume the leader role as an associate degree nurse?
3. Can you identify a role model who you feel is a good nurse leader? What qualities does he or she possess that makes him or her

a good nurse leader in your eyes? How could you incorporate these positive qualities into your own practice?

REFERENCES

Asselin, M. (2001). Time to wear a third hat? *Nursing Management, 32*(3), 24–28.

Brandt, M., Holt, J., & Sullivan, M. (2001). How to make conflict work for you. *Nursing Management, 32*(11), 32–35.

Ellis, J., & Hartley, C. (2003). *Nursing in today's world: Trends, issues, and management.* Philadelphia: Lippincott Williams & Wilkins.

Epstein, C. (1982).*The nurse leader: Philosophy and practice.* Reston, VA: Reston.

Gardner, J. (1990). *On leadership.* New York: Free Press.

Gardner, J. (n.d.). Tasks of leadership. Retrieved June 5, 2002, from http://www.leader-values.com

Gregory-Dawes, B. (2000). Changing times, changing roles. *AORN Journal, 72*(2), 177–178.

Kearney, R. (2001). *Advancing your career: Concepts of professional nursing.* Philadelphia: F.A. Davis.

Kerfoot, K. (1998). Leading change is leading creativity. *Dermatology Nursing, 10*(2), 142–144.

Mintzberg, H. (1975). The manager's job: Folklore and fact. *Harvard Business Review, 53,* 49–61.

Morgan, B. (2000). Testing leadership and management concepts: The relevancy factor. *Nurse Educator, 25*(4), 181–185.

Rost, J. (1994). Leadership: A new conception. *Holistic Nursing Practice, 9,* 1–8.

Wheatley, M. (1992). *Leadership and the new science learning about organizations from an orderly universe.* San Francisco: Berrett-Koehler.

SUGGESTED RESOURCES

Douglas, L. (1996). *The effective nurse: Leader and manager* (5th ed.). St. Louis, MO: Mosby.

Hood, L., & Leddy, S. (2002). *Leddy and Pepper's conceptual bases of professional nursing* (5th ed.). Philadelphia: Lippincott Williams & Wilkins.

Swansburg, R., & Swansburg, R. (2002). Introduction to management and leadership for nurse managers (3rd ed.). Sudbury, MA: Jones & Bartlett Publishers.

Tappen, R., Weiss, S., & Whitehead, D. (2001). *Essentials of nursing leadership and management* (3rd ed.). Philadelphia: F.A. Davis.

Chapter 9
Managing Client Care

▼ ▼ ▼ ▼ ▼ ▼ ▼

LEARNING OBJECTIVES

By the end of this chapter, you should be able to:

1. Identify ways to manage your clinical time effectively.
2. Relate methods to respond to and solve conflicts.
3. Identify methods to improve clinical decision making.
4. Identify ways to use resources appropriately.

KEY TERMS

Conflict
Conflict resolution
Resources
Time management

SCENARIO

Ling, a new RN, feels overwhelmed by her assignment on the medical-surgical floor. The floor has been very busy this shift. She is preparing to change the surgical dressing in Room 202. When she enters the room, she realizes that she forgot to bring tape and leaves to retrieve it. Once she uncovers the wound, she realizes that she did not bring enough dressings with her and must obtain more. While she is changing the dressing, the client contaminates the sterile field and Ling must get more supplies to complete the procedure. Ling feels frustrated that "everything I do today seems to go wrong." To make the situation worse, one of Ling's co-workers is reading a magazine while everyone is busy. Ling informs the co-worker, "It might be nice to have some help around here!"

*T*HINK ABOUT IT

1. Can you recall a day when each procedure seemed to take you twice as long as it should? Reflecting on the situation, does it seem that the delays were the result of a lack of organization?
2. Do you usually have a plan in mind when you approach a particular activity?
3. Identify someone who you feel is good at performing her job in a high-quality and timely manner. What organizational skills does this person display?

*I*NTRODUCTION

We will discuss the tasks of effectively managing time, conflicts, decisions, and resources in this chapter. Nursing is a job that involves human beings with a variety of needs and values. As an LPN, you have probably dealt with each of the above-mentioned tasks to at least some degree. As an associate degree prepared nurse, your role will change as you deal with each of these tasks. As an RN, you may be in charge of mentoring a team of caregivers and be responsible for time management, conflict management, decision making, and managing resources. Each of these tasks, if handled competently, will provide a more efficient and effective work environment.

*M*ANAGING TIME ON THE CLINICAL UNIT

Each of us views time from our own personal perspective of values, ideals, beliefs, and experiences.

Each of us views time from our own personal perspective of values, ideals, beliefs, and experiences. Some people have a relaxed view of time and amble through life. Some are always trying to beat the clock and slide in under the wire. Others approach time in a more organized, matter-of-fact manner, calculating how each minute can be utilized to the fullest. How we view time depends on whether we see time as rigid and exacting or flexible and free.

CRITICAL THINKING ACTIVITY

1. How do you view time?

_____

_____

_____

2. How does your view of time affect how you live and work?

_____

_____

_____

Time management is productively performing tasks in an organized, efficient manner.

As nurses, our daily schedules are generally packed as soon as we arrive on the job, especially now with the nursing shortage. Daily, we have more to do than we can comprehend accomplishing. Through the years nursing has developed many methods to improve workload organization, such as daily planning sheets, client kardexes, chart dividers, functional health patterns, and computer-generated flowcharts. Yet time management is a constant struggle.

In view of time management, do you take a minute to fluff a suffering client's pillow, or document a dressing change and attempt to stay somewhat on schedule? Do you offer a sip of water to a thirsty client, or grab a snack for break? Do you talk to a distressed client, or rush off to a committee meeting?

Time management is productively performing tasks in an organized, efficient manner. Writing down a schedule or list is part of time management. It gives direction and serves as a visual reference point throughout the day. Daily planning sheets help nurses plan their days. When you are first starting in a clinical setting, place all routine items on the daily planning sheet (Figure 9–1). Include such things as vital signs, treatments, medication administration, bathing the client, charting, and shift report. Only by listing all activities can you truly see the complete day. Refer to the planning sheet frequently throughout the day. Crossing off completed items gives a sense of progress and prevents errors and omissions. By placing treatments in designated time sections on the planning sheets, nurses are able to determine priorities and plan needed activities appropriately. As your organizational skills improve, you can omit some routine activities from the sheet. However, it is important that we not become so focused on individual procedures that we lose the holistic view of our client's needs.

Client	0700	0800	0900	1000	1100	1200	1300	1400	1500

Figure 9–1 Daily planning sheet.

To assist with organizational skills, complete a time log.

CRITICAL THINKING ACTIVITIES

1. Design your own daily planning sheet to help you be more organized. It could include a separate column or space for intravenous fluids, diet, intake and output, and so forth. Be creative. Share this with your classmates.

2. Discuss what the authors mean by the statement "it is important that we not become so focused on individual procedures that we lose the holistic view of our client's needs."

_____

_____

_____

If you are struggling with your organizational skills, it is a good idea to arrive a few minutes early to organize the day's planning sheets before your shift begins. Another tip to assist with organizational skills is to complete a time log. Use the daily planners discussed in Chapter 1 for three to seven days. Keep track of how you spend your time by listing everything you did in 15- or 30-minute segments. At the end of three days, analyze your schedule for items that could be deleted, combined, or revised. You may be surprised by how much time you spend on menial or insignificant tasks.

Some jobs or activities cannot be accomplished in a few minutes. You may need to set aside a block of time to prepare a report, analyze data, or prepare a time schedule.

3. Complete the following time log for three days.

Time	Activities	Time	Activities	Time	Activities
7:00		7:00		7:00	
7:30		7:30		7:30	
8:00		8:00		8:00	
8:30		8:30		8:30	
9:00		9:00		9:00	
9:30		9:30		9:30	
10:00		10:00		10:00	
10:30		10:30		10:30	
11:00		11:00		11:00	
11:30		11:30		11:30	
12:00		12:00		12:00	
12:30		12:30		12:30	
1:00		1:00		1:00	
1:30		1:30		1:30	

Time	Activities	Time	Activities	Time	Activities
2:00		2:00		2:00	
2:30		2:30		2:30	
3:00		3:00		3:00	
3:30		3:30		3:30	
4:00		4:00		4:00	
4:30		4:30		4:30	
5:00		5:00		5:00	
5:30		5:30		5:30	
6:00		6:00		6:00	
6:30		6:30		6:30	
7:00		7:00		7:00	
7:30		7:30		7:30	
8:00		8:00		8:00	
8:30		8:30		8:30	
9:00		9:00		9:00	
9:30		9:30		9:30	

4. After completing the time log, ask yourself these questions:

   • How have I wasted time?

   • Where have I duplicated activities?

   • What activities could have been combined?

   • Did I plan each day's activities? Did I follow my plan?

   • Did I complete priority items first each day?

   • What activities took longer than I thought they would? Why?

   • How could I revise my time log or my schedule to use my time more efficiently?

Monitor your schedule periodically to see how effectively you are using your time.

Nurses should continually analyze their work for duplication and repetition of duties. Tasks are often routinely performed without evaluating whether the task could be done differently to save time, whether it could be appropriately delegated, or whether the task needs to be done at all. Consider obtaining supplies for the next few planned treatments rather than obtaining supplies for one treatment at a time. Obtaining all the needed supplies will save time and eliminate unnecessary trips to the supply room. Review activities to see if you can complete more than one task at a time. Document a procedure immediately when it is completed so that the chart or computer is not handled multiple times. Plan ahead, and allow a buffer zone to complete tasks in case an emergency occurs. Using these time-saving tips will help you utilize your time more effectively. Monitor your schedule periodically to see how effectively you are using your time.

Personal ambition, drive, job requirements, and future goals often get in the way of our ability to say no when asked to serve on a committee or work an extended or second shift. Some nurses have such a need to be needed or wanted that saying no is very difficult for them. It is all right to say no. If your personal schedule is packed, or if the goals and plans of the committee do not interest you, learn to say no politely. Each of us needs time to replenish our souls to be productive and enjoy work. As you attempt to utilize your time more effectively, remember to save time for relaxation and personal endeavors. Include time to take walks in the park, meet a friend for lunch, see a funny movie, or attend a worship service.

CRITICAL THINKING ACTIVITIES

1. Complete the time assessment tool. When you completed your time log, did the results surprise you?

   _____

   _____

   _____

2. Using suggestions presented in the text and your own creativity, review your clinical experience this week and identify ways you could use your time more effectively. Write observations of your time management.

   _____

   _____

   _____

MANAGING CONFLICT

Conflict is a complex situation in which two parties have opposing views that may interfere with one of the two parties' reaching the desired goal.

Conflict is a complex situation in which two parties have opposing views that may interfere with one of the two parties' reaching the desired goal. Conflict is multidimensional, stemming from varying values, beliefs, attitudes, and cultures. Conflict is often avoided. Most people do not desire or seek conflict. Rarely is conflict seen as a welcome occasion to grow, an opportunity to expand horizons, or a chance to produce a change. However, conflict handled productively can produce growth and constructive change. A challenge for all of us is to change our view of conflict. Effective conflict management is an essential learned skill. It is imperative that nurses learn to handle conflict constructively to provide quality client care. If a nurse has to work in an environment of constant conflict, she cannot effectively concentrate on client needs and care. Bartol, Parrish, and McSweeney (2001) state, "Ineffective intervention can lower employee morale, decrease productivity, increase absenteeism and turnover, foster resistance to change, and interfere with employee development" (p. 35). Therefore, it is essential that we learn to handle conflict in a mature, positive manner.

Identifying Personal Attitudes toward Conflict

Identifying your attitude toward conflict and your usual method of handling conflict is the first step toward effectively handling conflict. Bartol and McSweeney's Conflict Management Scale, which is based on the ideas of Hall (1973), measures attitude toward managing conflict (Bartol, 1976). This tool is reproduced in Figure 9–2 and can be useful in determining your approach to conflict.

CRITICAL THINKING ACTIVITY

1. Complete the Bartol and McSweeney Conflict Management Scale. According to this assessment tool, what is your style for handling conflict?

_____

_____

_____

The five styles of handling conflict are collaborative, compromise, accommodative, forcing, and avoidance.

According to Hall's ideas on conflict, there are five methods or styles of handling conflict as it relates to concern for relationships and concern for attaining goals. The five styles of handling conflict are *collaborative, compromise, accommodative, forcing,* and *avoidance.* The collaborative style values relationships and goals. A person with a collaborative style approaches a situation in a manner that seeks to creatively solve the problem with the belief that the process of working through the problem will strengthen relationships.

BARTOL/McSWEENEY CONFLICT MANAGEMENT SCALE

DIRECTIONS: Please darken in the space to the right of each statement that most closely indicates the extent to which you agree or disagree that the statement reflects your style of managing interpersonal conflict. Please respond to all items.

1 = Strongly agree   2 = Agree   3 = Disagree   4 = Strongly disagree

	❏ 1	❏ 2	❏ 3	❏ 4
1. It is important to recognize tension in relationships and confront the difficulty if problems are to be solved.	❏ 1	❏ 2	❏ 3	❏ 4
2. I give in for the sake of the common good, knowing I will get another chance later.	❏ 1	❏ 2	❏ 3	❏ 4
3. When conflict is honestly admitted and accurately interpreted, relationships can be strengthened.	❏ 1	❏ 2	❏ 3	❏ 4
4. I stick to the rules to avoid disagreements because I can't be bothered with arguments.	❏ 1	❏ 2	❏ 3	❏ 4
5. Compromise can be reached if extreme positions are eliminated by negotiation.	❏ 1	❏ 2	❏ 3	❏ 4
6. Attempts to resolve conflicts are fruitless in the long run; it is best to keep your distance.	❏ 1	❏ 2	❏ 3	❏ 4
7. I keep out of the way when I see disagreements among my co-workers; one needs to learn to sidestep conflict.	❏ 1	❏ 2	❏ 3	❏ 4
8. There is no room for hesitancy or doubt in conflict resolution or others may see you as wishy-washy.	❏ 1	❏ 2	❏ 3	❏ 4
9. It is better to sacrifice your goals than to threaten a relationship.	❏ 1	❏ 2	❏ 3	❏ 4
10. All is fair when you believe your goal is the correct one.	❏ 1	❏ 2	❏ 3	❏ 4
11. Progress through compromise is the best way to resolve conflict.	❏ 1	❏ 2	❏ 3	❏ 4
12. Arguing is futile, silence can be eloquent and helps you avoid trouble.	❏ 1	❏ 2	❏ 3	❏ 4
13. I overlook others' shortcomings for the sake of maintaining relationships and keeping peace.	❏ 1	❏ 2	❏ 3	❏ 4
14. I let things ride rather than risk causing irreparable damage to a relationship.	❏ 1	❏ 2	❏ 3	❏ 4
15. I worry when I have a disagreement with another because I don't want to create divisions.	❏ 1	❏ 2	❏ 3	❏ 4
16. I try to encourage brainstorming when differences arise. Many ideas are explored and often I am pleasantly surprised at the results.	❏ 1	❏ 2	❏ 3	❏ 4
17. It is better to remain aloof and disengaged than to get involved in useless discussion when there is disagreement.	❏ 1	❏ 2	❏ 3	❏ 4
18. People should face the fact that there is only one correct way to do things.	❏ 1	❏ 2	❏ 3	❏ 4
19. I will give in a little in the beginning if it affords me an opportunity to get something else later.	❏ 1	❏ 2	❏ 3	❏ 4
20. I am careful not to step on another's toes; no idea is worth destroying a relationship.	❏ 1	❏ 2	❏ 3	❏ 4

Figure 9–2 Bartol/McSweeney Conflict Management Scale.

1 = Strongly agree   2 = Agree   3 = Disagree   4 = Strongly disagree

21. I talk about differences openly in an effort to resolve possible underlying ❑ 1   ❑ 2   ❑ 3   ❑ 4
    conflict before taking any actions.

22. I feel insecure when someone disagrees with me because I am afraid ❑ 1   ❑ 2   ❑ 3   ❑ 4
    that means I am disliked.

23. I try to encourage the expression of what underlies conflict; it helps all ❑ 1   ❑ 2   ❑ 3   ❑ 4
    parties to be aware of the problems.

24. The only sensible thing to do when there is conflict is to simply ❑ 1   ❑ 2   ❑ 3   ❑ 4
    withdraw and wait for things to blow over.

25. Conflict may be a sign of incomplete understanding, or hidden ❑ 1   ❑ 2   ❑ 3   ❑ 4
    personal feelings. The underlying causes can only be discovered through
    honest discussion.

26. Exploration and discussion of differing viewpoints lays the groundwork ❑ 1   ❑ 2   ❑ 3   ❑ 4
    for creative resolution of conflict.

27. Avoiding arguments is important to me because I've learned discussion ❑ 1   ❑ 2   ❑ 3   ❑ 4
    of different opinions gets you nowhere.

28. A problem-solving approach based on respect for other people and their ❑ 1   ❑ 2   ❑ 3   ❑ 4
    goals should characterize our approach to conflict.

29. Conflicts should not be explored nor the underlying tensions identified; ❑ 1   ❑ 2   ❑ 3   ❑ 4
    avoidance is the best course.

30. Whenever there is conflict it is the best team that wins, and that is ❑ 1   ❑ 2   ❑ 3   ❑ 4
    how it should be.

31. When there is disagreement, I call attention to that fact and suggest ❑ 1   ❑ 2   ❑ 3   ❑ 4
    that we explore the needs and opinions of everyone involved.

32. When there is conflict, I am curious about how others are thinking and ❑ 1   ❑ 2   ❑ 3   ❑ 4
    feeling, and concerned with getting everything out into the open that
    needs to be.

33. Indifference is the best shield in conflict; in that way you can sidestep ❑ 1   ❑ 2   ❑ 3   ❑ 4
    the problem.

34. I give in to others on lesser points and try to win what is more important ❑ 1   ❑ 2   ❑ 3   ❑ 4
    to me.

35. When there is a disagreement with others, I suggest we discuss our ❑ 1   ❑ 2   ❑ 3   ❑ 4
    differences. Closer relationships and creative solutions are often
    the result.

36. I would forget my goals rather than risk displeasing a friend. ❑ 1   ❑ 2   ❑ 3   ❑ 4

37. When there is conflict, I try to open it up so that every aspect of people's ❑ 1   ❑ 2   ❑ 3   ❑ 4
    feelings and the issue at hand gets thoroughly considered.

38. When there is conflict, I am interested in knowing what others are ❑ 1   ❑ 2   ❑ 3   ❑ 4
    thinking and feeling; getting everything out into the open that needs
    to be.

39. When there is a disagreement the minority should give into the ❑ 1   ❑ 2   ❑ 3   ❑ 4
    majority so progress can be made. Everyone gets their chance.

40. The underlying reasons for conflict can only be discovered through ❑ 1   ❑ 2   ❑ 3   ❑ 4
    candid and objective discussion.

Figure 9–2 (continued)

1 = Strongly agree   2 = Agree   3 = Disagree   4 = Strongly disagree

41. Sometimes it is necessary to give into others if progress is to be made. ❏ 1   ❏ 2   ❏ 3   ❏ 4
You will get another chance later.

42. You can't win all the time; good sportsmanship requires compromise. ❏ 1   ❏ 2   ❏ 3   ❏ 4

43. Personal relationships are more important than achieving personal goals. ❏ 1   ❏ 2   ❏ 3   ❏ 4

44. It is unrealistic to think you can always win; you should expect to   ❏ 1   ❏ 2   ❏ 3   ❏ 4
compromise on some points.

45. I owe it to myself to accomplish what I set out to do, regardless of   ❏ 1   ❏ 2   ❏ 3   ❏ 4
whose feelings get hurt.

46. Impersonal tolerance is the most enlightened approach to handling   ❏ 1   ❏ 2   ❏ 3   ❏ 4
conflict and the best way to avoid trouble.

47. It is better to go along with others than to provoke antagonism.   ❏ 1   ❏ 2   ❏ 3   ❏ 4

48. Conflicts are a necessary evil, but I have learned to dodge them and   ❏ 1   ❏ 2   ❏ 3   ❏ 4
avoid involvement.

49. One must guard against causing irreparable damage to a relationship   ❏ 1   ❏ 2   ❏ 3   ❏ 4
just to achieve some goal.

50. Maintaining good interpersonal relationships is more important than   ❏ 1   ❏ 2   ❏ 3   ❏ 4
achieving personal goals.

51. The only sensible thing to do when there is conflict is to wait it out.   ❏ 1   ❏ 2   ❏ 3   ❏ 4

52. I would lay my personal goals aside before I would jeopardize   ❏ 1   ❏ 2   ❏ 3   ❏ 4
a relationship.

53. Keeping your distance is the best policy when you see a conflict   ❏ 1   ❏ 2   ❏ 3   ❏ 4
developing.

54. Conflict requires self-sacrifice and placing the importance of continued   ❏ 1   ❏ 2   ❏ 3   ❏ 4
relationship above one's own goals.

55. I owe it to myself to prevail in conflicts with others whose goals   ❏ 1   ❏ 2   ❏ 3   ❏ 4
are different.

56. In disagreements with others, I owe it to myself to avoid any pressure   ❏ 1   ❏ 2   ❏ 3   ❏ 4
to compromise.

57. Power, and even force may be used when your goal is important to you.   ❏ 1   ❏ 2   ❏ 3   ❏ 4

58. Survival of the fittest applied to human relations is a basic test of   ❏ 1   ❏ 2   ❏ 3   ❏ 4
one's ability to deal effectively with conflict.

59. You never get anywhere if you give in to others when there is a   ❏ 1   ❏ 2   ❏ 3   ❏ 4
disagreement about goals.

60. I avoid calling attention to disagreements with the hope they will   ❏ 1   ❏ 2   ❏ 3   ❏ 4
just disappear.

61. Conflicts should be explored and the underlying tensions identified if   ❏ 1   ❏ 2   ❏ 3   ❏ 4
problem solving is to be successful.

62. Exploration and discussion of conflict leads to creative resolution   ❏ 1   ❏ 2   ❏ 3   ❏ 4
of conflict.

63. I find conflict disturbing so I give in readily to others and try to keep   ❏ 1   ❏ 2   ❏ 3   ❏ 4
everyone happy.

64. It is a fact of life, some people are right and some are wrong; I aim to   ❏ 1   ❏ 2   ❏ 3   ❏ 4
win regardless.

Figure 9–2 (continued)

1 = Strongly agree   2 = Agree   3 = Disagree   4 = Strongly disagree

65. I am willing to bargain and negotiate to preserve the common good.	❏ 1	❏ 2	❏ 3	❏ 4
66. I prefer to walk away when I see an argument is starting.	❏ 1	❏ 2	❏ 3	❏ 4
67. Arguments should be avoided because they only drive people apart.	❏ 1	❏ 2	❏ 3	❏ 4
68. I won't reveal any hesitancy or doubt when I become involved in a disagreement, because it may be seen as a sign of weakness.	❏ 1	❏ 2	❏ 3	❏ 4
69. When there is a disagreement I prefer to wait it out rather than become involved in useless discussion.	❏ 1	❏ 2	❏ 3	❏ 4
70. Persuasion, power, and even force are all acceptable ways to resolve a conflict.	❏ 1	❏ 2	❏ 3	❏ 4
71. I enjoy using my skills and persuasive ability to maneuver toward my goals when there is conflict.	❏ 1	❏ 2	❏ 3	❏ 4

(Printed with permission of Dr. Bartol and Dr. McSweeney.)

Figure 9–2 (continued)

In the compromise style, an individual approaches the problem believing she can use persuasive influence to sway or convince the group to choose a certain option and put aside personal desires for the good of the group. By considering the interests of the group, relationships are maintained. All group members are encouraged to express personal opinions and views. The basic belief is that everyone will win sometimes.

The accommodative style views relationships as most important. An accommodative person willingly releases her goals for the sake of the relationship. She avoids conflict at all costs.

The forcing style centers on the goal and forsakes the relationship. An individual with a forcing style uses confidence, firmness, power, and force to obtain the goal. Others' desires are forced aside.

In the avoidance style, the individual ignores personal goals and does not value relationships. This person expects to lose in conflicts, so she avoids all issues that approach conflict and becomes detached in such situations. She sees energy spent on resolving conflict as wasted, especially because the individual will not win anyway.

By imagining each of these individuals approaching a conflict, we can see how our view of conflict directly influences how we resolve conflict. If we change our view of conflict we can approach the situation more

SAMPLE OF COMPLETED HAND SCORE SHEET - CONFLICT MANAGEMENT

ID# _____

Place the numeral (1, 2, 3, or 4) corresponding to your choice next to the number of the item on the score sheet. Then, total the numerals you chose in each column and write the total in the space provided. Last, divide the total by the number of items in each column. For example, divide the total in the collaborative column by 16 and by 11 in the compromise, etc. The lowest score represents your preferred conflict management style. The next lowest score, your second choice, etc. The five scores will show your pattern of managing conflict.

Collaborative	Compromise	Accomodative	Forcing	Avoidant
_1_ 1	_2_ 2	_3_ 9	_4_ 8	_1_ 4
_3_ 3	_2_ 5	_3_ 13	_4_ 10	_2_ 6
_3_ 16	_3_ 11	_4_ 14	_4_ 18	_1_ 7
_4_ 21	_2_ 19	_2_ 15	_3_ 30	_2_ 12
_3_ 23	_2_ 34	_2_ 20	_4_ 45	_2_ 17
_2_ 25	_2_ 39	_3_ 22	_4_ 55	_3_ 24
_2_ 26	_2_ 41	_4_ 36	_3_ 56	_2_ 27
_2_ 28	_1_ 42	_2_ 43	_4_ 57	_3_ 29
_3_ 31	_1_ 44	_3_ 47	_3_ 58	_1_ 33
_2_ 32	_2_ 65	_3_ 49	_3_ 59	_2_ 46
_4_ 35	_3_ 71	_2_ 50	_4_ 64	_1_ 48
_3_ 37		_3_ 52	_3_ 68	_3_ 51
_3_ 38		_3_ 54	_4_ 70	_1_ 53
_4_ 40		_3_ 63		_1_ 60
_1_ 61				_1_ 66
_3_ 62				_2_ 67
				_1_ 69

Total Columns _43_ Total   _22_ Total   _40_ Total   _47_ Total   _29_ Total

Divide by   16   11   14   13   17

Final Score   _2.69_   _2.00_   _2.86_   _3.62_   _1.71_

1. *Preferred Choice - Avoidant*
Pattern of back-up choices
2. *Compromise   3. Collaborative   4. Accomodative*
Least Preferred - Forcing

Figure 9–2 (continued)

HAND SCORE SHEET - CONFLICT MANAGEMENT

ID# _____

Place the numeral (1, 2, 3, or 4) corresponding to your choice next to the number of the item on the score sheet. Then, total the numerals you chose in each column and write the total in the space provided. Last, divide the total by the number of items in each column. For example, divide the total in the collaborative column by 16 and by 11 in the compromise, etc. The lowest score represents your preferred conflict management style. The next lowest score, your second choice, etc. The five scores will show your pattern of managing conflict.

Collaborative	Compromise	Accomodative	Forcing	Avoidant
___ 1	___ 2	___ 9	___ 8	___ 4
___ 3	___ 5	___ 13	___ 10	___ 6
___ 16	___ 11	___ 14	___ 18	___ 7
___ 21	___ 19	___ 15	___ 30	___ 12
___ 23	___ 34	___ 20	___ 45	___ 17
___ 25	___ 39	___ 22	___ 55	___ 24
___ 26	___ 41	___ 36	___ 56	___ 27
___ 28	___ 42	___ 43	___ 57	___ 29
___ 31	___ 44	___ 47	___ 58	___ 33
___ 32	___ 65	___ 49	___ 59	___ 46
___ 35	___ 71	___ 50	___ 64	___ 48
___ 37		___ 52	___ 68	___ 51
___ 38		___ 54	___ 70	___ 53
___ 40		___ 63		___ 60
___ 61				___ 66
___ 62				___ 67
				___ 69

Total Columns ___ Total   ___ Total   ___ Total   ___ Total   ___ Total

Divide by   16   11   14   13   17

Final Score _____   _____   _____   _____   _____

Figure 9–2 (continued)

objectively and confidently. We can move more creatively and productively toward a collaborative approach where goals and relationships can be preserved and maintained.

Sources of Conflict

Some sources of conflict are personal conflicts, role definition, resources, group conflict, and workload.

In the health field, various cultures, genders, socioeconomic groups, and educational levels are brought together. Each individual in these groups approaches a situation a little differently. Therein breeds conflict. Some sources of conflict are personal conflicts, role definition, resources, group conflict, and workload.

Personal Conflicts

Each person has different values and beliefs and, based on these, makes decisions. Thus each person approaches situations from a different angle based on personal values and beliefs and thinks her way is the best way to handle the problem. As these different approaches to solving the problem converge, conflict arises.

Role Definition

In times of nursing shortages and economic downturns, management requests individuals to assume multiple roles. Sometimes these roles overlap or are not well defined, and confusion arises as to who is to perform what role. This can lead to role conflict.

Resources

As people scramble for limited supplies, pay raises, equipment, and personnel, conflict can occur because each person or department wants her or its share of the pie. This is especially likely to occur when resources are at a premium.

Group Conflicts

Each individual belongs to a variety of group types, such as gender, occupation, culture, and role. Two groups may disagree and conflict with each other. Conflicts over wages and job assignments may occur. Nurses may disagree with an administrative decision. For example, consider nurses who have worked at a facility for several years at one pay level and newly hired nurses with less experience who start at a higher or equal pay level. The issue causes conflict between the groups.

Workload

In times of nursing shortages, workloads may increase. Some individuals may not mind the overload if it means more pay, while others desire more personal time more than the extra money. Increased workloads also make employees tired, and tensions increase when personal resources are exhausted.

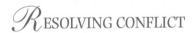ESOLVING CONFLICT

Conflict resolution is not about winning or losing.

Resolving conflict is not like a boxing match in which one person or group is knocked out and the other one wins with a few bruises. Conflict resolution is not about winning or losing. Instead, **conflict resolution** is two individuals or groups working effectively together to come to an agreement both can accept. In this way, no one is a winner who must stay on top and watch for the next battle. No one is a loser who wastes energy plotting the next round in a disagreement. Nor is there a tie leading to a stalemate with no resolution to the issue.

When conflict arises there are strategies that you can use to resolve the situation effectively. Consider the following ideas on effective conflict resolution:

1. Concentrate on issues, not on individual personalities.
2. Claim responsibility for personal involvement where appropriate.
3. Communicate openly and assertively without aggression.
4. Listen attentively to the other's statements and concerns.
5. Creatively look for commonalities and solutions.
6. Examine the consequences of each solution. (Zerwekh & Claborn, 2003)

Gottlieb and Healey (1990) present a practical process in solving conflict that includes identifying the source of conflict, generating possible solutions, examining suggested solutions, choosing the best solution, implementing the chosen solution and evaluating the effectiveness of the solution for the conflict, and deciding if the conflict has been resolved or if the conflict-solving process needs repeating.

Identifying the Source

Sometimes the source of conflict is obvious, and other times it is hidden in other agendas. Emotional involvement can color a person's objectivity, hiding the solution to the real problem of conflict. If the problem is not obvious, objectively discuss the situation to bring the problem into focus. It is important for all parties involved to attentively listen to one another's concerns until the source of conflict has been identified. Sometimes an objective third party can help identify the problem.

Generating Possible Solutions

During this solution generation phase it is important to state your personal desires for the solution to the conflict. It is also important to brainstorm during this phase. All potential solutions that come to mind should be presented even if they appear unconventional. Such suggestions can lead to a creative, satisfying solution that might otherwise have been overlooked.

Examining Suggested Solutions

Once all solutions have been presented, open-mindedly and impartially review them and evaluate which solution or solutions might work. Evaluate the suggested solutions without considering who made the suggestions. Sometimes a suggestion may be rejected because of personal status or personal feelings about the person who made the suggestion. Be aware of personal feelings about others when examining possible solutions. Discuss these feelings as appropriate, but stay focused on the issues, not personalities. During the problem-solving process it is important to be flexible.

Choosing the Best Solution

If each step of the conflict resolution process is followed and given adequate time for solution emergence, creative solutions are identified and the end product is an effective, quality solution to a puzzling conflict.

After carefully considering the ramifications of all suggested options, chose the best solution to appropriately resolve the conflict. Sometimes by combining several suggestions a more creative and satisfying solution is obtained.

Implementing the Chosen Solution and Evaluating Its Effectiveness

Once the solution has been implemented, choose a date to evaluate the results. The implemented solution needs an appropriate amount of time to be effective. Aborting the process before allowing adequate implementation time may be unfair to the solution and to the parties involved.

Deciding if the Conflict Has Been Resolved

If the solution does not work and the conflict is not resolved, the process of resolving the conflict needs to be repeated. Perhaps the real issue was not identified in the first attempt. Spend time discussing the conflict further to truly identify the issue. Conflict resolution takes time and energy. If each step of the conflict resolution process is followed and given adequate time for solution emergence, creative solutions are identified and the end product is an effective, quality solution to a puzzling conflict. Conflict can be a growth process.

CRITICAL THINKING ACTIVITIES

1. Analyze the advantages and disadvantages of each step of Zerwekh and Claborn's conflict resolution (2003).

Conflict Style	Advantages	Disadvantages
• Concentrate on issues, not on individual personalities.	_____	_____
• Claim responsibility for personal involvement where appropriate.	_____	_____
• Communicate openly and assertively without aggression.	_____	_____
• Listen attentively to the other's statements and concerns.	_____	_____
• Creatively look for commonalities and solutions.	_____	_____
• Examine the consequences of each solution.	_____	_____

2. How have your thoughts about conflict been challenged or changed after reading this section?

_____

_____

_____

$\mathcal{M}$ANAGING DECISIONS

In the clinical setting, you need to make quick, accurate decisions regarding the clients assigned to your care.

In Chapter 5 we discussed clinical judgment, problem solving, decision making, and the nursing process. In the clinical setting, you need to make quick, accurate decisions regarding the clients assigned to your care. Your client's future is determined by the clinical decisions you make. It is a sobering thought that "patient's lives hang in the balance of skilled nursing judgment" (Tanner, 2000, p. 338).

Faculty members are constantly attempting to find methods to assist students in making the leap from theory to clinical judgments. Your faculty members encourage you to think critically and creatively in your classroom discussions and clinical experiences. They may use various methods to encourage critical thinking, such as case studies/scenarios, computer-simulated clinical experiences, and journaling. Classroom discussions and written case studies or scenarios do not replace the clinical experience of working with a client needing immediate, appropriate, therapeutic nursing action. "Written scenarios may not capture the unpredictable, dynamic, moment-to-moment reasoning of nursing practice" (Fowler, 1997, p. 350). According to a research study by Fowler, "experiential knowledge is a component of clinical reasoning" (p. 361). Knowledge gained and applied in a clinical situation assists us in making decisions and determining decisive, appropriate nursing actions.

"Clinical decision making is a problem-solving activity that focuses on defining patient problems and selecting appropriate treatment interventions" (Higuchi & Donald, 2002, p. 145). Higuchi and Donald describe six thinking processes that nurses use in clinical decision making: *description, selection, inference, hypothesizing, synthesis,* and *verification*.

Description is the listing of facts as they relate to the client, for example, the findings of a client assessment such as vital signs, breath sounds, heart sounds, and so forth. Nurses also describe the nursing action they are taking to meet the client's needs.

Selection is choosing relevant data or information about the client to report or chart. The nurse must know the data to collect and must sort out the relevant, important data to report. Selection as a thinking skill requires knowledge from theory and critical decision-making abilities. Skill in making decisions can be gained and improved by following the decision-making process described in Chapter 5.

Inference includes three thinking functions: categorizing, discovering relationships among the separate parts, and hypothesizing. A nurse with sound clinical judgment is able to place appropriate data in different categories or sections so the data can be documented and communicated in an effective way. An example of categorizing would be placing data relating to the heart in one category and data relating to the renal system in another category. The nurse needs knowledge to know what data to collect and needs nursing judgment to review the data as a unit. To discover the relationship between these separate parts, the nurse would review the data in the cardiac system and the data in the renal system and then discover how the renal function is affecting the heart and how the heart is affecting the renal function. The conclusion the nurse drew from the data she reviewed would be her hypothesis, or assumption; for example, she could hypothesize that the kidneys are not producing enough urine because the heart cannot adequately pump the blood through the body to the renal system.

Synthesis is combining the separate parts of a whole and determining a nursing action; for example, after obtaining and reviewing cardiac, renal, and respiratory system data, the nurse determines that the client with congestive heart failure needs oxygen. "The ability to intuitively grasp a situation as a whole is one of the characteristics of nursing expertise" (Higuchi & Donald, 2002, p. 151).

Verification is assessing data as valid and asserting appropriate results. Nurses verify data by documenting it and asserting the nursing action taken as appropriate. In our congestive heart failure example, verification is the nurse's documenting assessment data after starting oxygen that confirms appropriate nursing action occurred to improve client status.

Every day, nurses use description, selection, inference, hypothesizing, synthesis, and verification in the clinical setting. Use the following critical thinking activity to evaluate your clinical thinking skills.

CRITICAL THINKING ACTIVITY

1. Review your clinical experiences over the past few weeks and describe examples of each of the thinking processes you have used in making clinical decisions.

   • Description:

   _____

   _____

   _____

   • Selection:

   _____

   _____

   _____

- Inference (include examples of categorizing, discovering relationships among the separate parts, and hypothesizing):

_____

_____

_____

- Synthesis:

_____

_____

_____

- Verification:

_____

_____

_____

$\mathcal{M}$ANAGING RESOURCES

Resources are usable commodities available to meet a need.

Resources are usable commodities available to meet a need. These resources include personnel, equipment, supplies, and finances. All of these must be managed and utilized effectively to provide quality client care. In times of an economic downturn, resources are distributed sparingly.

Wise use of personnel is especially important to improve job satisfaction, prevent burnout, and provide sufficient nurse-client ratios. Providing an encouraging, supportive, nonthreatening environment for nursing personnel is one of the best ways to care for the resource of personnel.

Facility resources should include a convenient layout to prevent wasted time and energy. It is important to have and maintain state-of-the-art equipment, quality client care, accurate diagnoses, and time-saving devices. Continuing education provides staff with updated education. Nurses can do their jobs more efficiently with assistance from members of the ancillary team such as housekeeping, pastoral care, and volunteer services. Ideally, if available resources are used wisely, overhead is decreased, needed resources are purchased, and nursing salaries increased.

CRITICAL THINKING ACTIVITY

1. What are some ways you could use your facility's resources more productively?

_____

_____

_____

$\mathcal{S}$UMMARY

Job satisfaction improves when we learn to manage time, conflict, decisions, and resources.

Job satisfaction improves when we learn to manage time, conflict, decisions, and resources. Wise use of time provides quality client care, excellent job performance, and valuable self-care. We can enjoy our work more fully when we realize that conflict will occur and that it does not have to be viewed as a battleground but, rather, as an opportunity for change and growth. Your self-confidence in the workplace will improve as you learn to make effective, sound decisions. These sound decisions will allow you to provide safe and competent care to your clients. Increased self-confidence while caring for your clients can be comforting to them and ease their anxieties, leading to a more pleasant healing process. Wise use of resources provides an adequate quantity of supplies and improved fiscal security. Knowing and understanding these concepts related to managing client care can and will prove valuable to you as you move ahead in your career.

$\mathcal{C}$HAPTER REFLECTIONS

Looking back on the opening scenario in this chapter, answer the following questions:

1. What was going on in this scenario that made Ling frustrated?
2. What could Ling do to manage her time more appropriately?
3. What is the source of the conflict between the co-workers?
4. What more effective approach could Ling have taken with her co-worker to obtain assistance?

REFERENCES

Bartol, G. (1976). *The styles of conflict management used in co-worker relationships by nurse practitioners employed in hospitals.* Unpublished doctoral dissertation, Teachers College, Columbia University.

Bartol, G., Parrish, R., & McSweeney, M. (2001). Effective conflict management begins with knowing your style. *Journal for Nurses in Staff Development, 17*(1), 34–40.

Fowler, L. (1997). Clinical reasoning strategies used during care planning. *Clinical Nursing Research, 6*(4), 349–362.

Gottlieb, M., & Healy, W. (1990). *Making deals: The business of negotiating.* New York: New York Institute of Finance.

Hall, J. (1973). *Conflict management survey.* Conroe, TX: Telemetric International.

Higuchi, K., & Donald, J. (2002). Thinking processes used by nurses in clinical decision-making. *Journal of Nursing Education, 41*(4), 145–155.

Tanner, C. (2000). Critical thinking: Beyond nursing process. *Journal of Nursing Education, 39*(8), 338 [On-line]. Available: http://80-proquest.umi.com

Zerwekh, J., & Claborn, J. (2003). *Nursing today: Transition and trends* (4th ed.). St. Louis: Saunders.

SUGGESTED RESOURCES

Asselin, M. (2001). Time to wear a third hat? *Nursing Management, 32*(3), 24–29.

Brandt, M., Holt, J., & Sullivan, M. (2001). How to make conflict work for you. *Nursing Management, 32*(11), 32–35.

Tappen, R., Weiss, S., & Whitehead, D. (2001). *Essentials of nursing leadership and management* (3rd ed.). Philadelphia: F.A. Davis.

Tomey, A. (2000). *Guide to nursing management and leadership* (6th ed.). St. Louis, MO: Mosby.

Valentine, P. (2001). A gender perspective on conflict management strategies of nurses. *Journal of Nursing Scholarship, 33*(1), 69–74.

Walczak, M., & Absolon, P. (2001). Essentials for effective communication in oncology nursing: Assertiveness, conflict management, delegation, and motivation. *Journal for Nurses in Staff Development, 17*(3), 159–162.

$\mathscr{P}$ART IV
Professional Considerations

▼ ▼ ▼ ▼ ▼ ▼ ▼

$\mathcal{C}$hapter 10
Nursing Theory as a
Basis to Practice Nursing

▼ ▼ ▼ ▼ ▼ ▼ ▼

$\mathcal{L}$EARNING OBJECTIVES

By the end of this chapter you should be able to:

1. Define nursing theory.
2. Identify major concepts in nursing.
3. Identify scientific theories that influence nursing theory.
4. Explain how nursing theory is a basis for nursing practice.
5. Examine the relationship of nursing theory, nursing research, and nursing practice.

$\mathcal{K}$EY TERMS

Concepts
Metaparadigm
Nursing concept
Nursing theorists
Nursing theory
Paradigms
Phenomena
Philosophy
Science
Theory
Validity
Variables

$\mathscr{S}$CENARIO

Kory is studying for a test and is wondering why theory is such a big deal in nursing. He feels that theory is of no use to the nurse working on the floor. After all, he has been an LPN for five years and has never had to use theory to give what he considers good care to his clients. Kory thinks that theory is "just something nurses with big degrees talk about using in practice." He has never heard anyone say that the facility is providing care in a particular manner because of a nursing theory or research studies.

$\mathscr{T}$HINK ABOUT IT

1. What do you think nursing theory is?
2. Are you familiar with any nursing theorists? If so, which ones?
3. Does your facility or your school of nursing follow a particular theorist? If so, which one?

$\mathscr{I}$NTRODUCTION

In this chapter we will discuss nursing theory and the major nursing concepts. We will explore the definition of nursing theory and how it defines nursing as a respected science, art, and profession. We will see how scientific theories influence nursing theory and how nursing theory and research influence and relate to nursing practice. Finally, we will look at the associate degree–prepared nurse's role in nursing theory and research with regard to nursing practice. What does nursing theory mean to you as you transition into your new role as an associate degree prepared RN?

$\mathscr{M}$AJOR CONCEPTS IN NURSING

Have you ever had an idea that would either make your nursing practice better or improve client care or outcomes? This type of idea can and does inspire nursing theory. An individual has an idea and then sets out to prove it in a systematic fashion. The development of a nursing theory leads to an increase in knowledge, research, and education for the practice of nursing and therefore an opportunity to provide better quality client care. Nursing theory is not a new concept. Florence

Nightingale, the first nursing theorist, developed her environmental theory during the Crimean War more than 140 years ago. In her 1859 *Notes on Nursing*, Nightingale identified factors that affected health and wellness and documented her beliefs with observations, statistics, and deductive reasoning (Kearney, 2001).

Nursing theory gives us a philosophy of what we believe and is the framework that guides nursing actions. A nursing theory helps provide supportive, researched data to improve nursing practice by describing, predicting, and controlling **phenomena** (Tomey & Alligood, 2002). A phenomenon is any fact or event that we can detect through the use of our senses. An example of a phenomenon is a nurse taking a blood pressure reading and detecting variations when the client is in different positions, such as sitting, standing, or lying down. A nurse can control the position, or phenomenon. **Nursing theory** consists of ideas that attempt to explain a relationship between two or more **concepts** (views or ideas about something). The concepts in the blood pressure illustration are the variations in the blood pressure with the different, controlled positions. Concepts are considered to be the subject matter or building blocks of nursing theory. These concepts or ideas are the labels given the phenomenon in question. They are ideas or mental images that originate in the mind of an individual or group of individuals from a particular experience that they have had in their nursing career. For example, when you turn an immobile client every two hours, you have the concept or idea that turning prevents the client from skin breakdown.

Concepts are said to be either *abstract* or *concrete*. Abstract concepts do not refer to a specific time or place and are sometimes defined as a mental image or picture. Concrete concepts relate to a particular time, place, or thing (Tomey & Alligood, 2002). A **nursing concept** is a concrete or abstract idea about nursing. Table 10–1 gives examples of abstract and concrete concepts as they apply to Nightingale's environmental theory.

Concepts may be referred to as **variables** when they are measured in research studies to develop a theory. The terms *measurable concept* and *variable* actually mean the same thing and are used interchangeably. An example of a measurable concept or variable is a client's blood pressure. You can measure a client's blood pressure and compare it to his blood pressure in different situations or in relation to different variables.

Table 10–1 Abstract and concrete concepts using Nightingale's environment theory

Abstract concepts	Concrete concepts
Environment	Ventilation
	Light
	Cleanliness
	Warmth
	Noise level
	Diet

CRITICAL THINKING ACTIVITIES

1. Share an idea you think would improve your nursing practice.

_____

_____

_____

2. Share examples of concepts that are measurable.

_____

_____

_____

Nursing theory exists to scientifically define and support the realm of nursing as a profession with its own body of knowledge.

When a relationship is assumed to exist between a set of variables, a theoretical statement is developed and then systematically tested. When the relationship between a set of variables is scientifically proven, and it is proven that the theoretical statement is applicable to nursing practice, it is recognized as a nursing theory.

Nursing theory exists to scientifically define and support the realm of nursing as a profession with its own body of knowledge. Perhaps the most abstract or general level of nursing knowledge is referred to as the **metaparadigm** of nursing. *Metaparadigm* is defined as the main phenomena of interest to a particular discipline. The main phenomena considered of interest to nursing center around the concepts *person, environment, health,* and *nursing.* These concepts are the universal tools that nursing theorists and nursing organizations use to write their individual philosophies of nursing. In addition, each person has his personal definition of what the concepts of the nursing metaparadigm mean to his own practice of nursing. For example, you may feel that health is the absence of illness. As you continue to practice in the field of nursing, your experiences will change your definition of what these concepts mean.

CRITICAL THINKING ACTIVITY

1. Write your personal definitions of the following concepts.
    *   Person:

    _____
    _____
    _____

    *   Environment:

    _____
    _____
    _____

    *   Health:

    _____
    _____
    _____

    *   Nursing:

    _____
    _____
    _____

Philosophy (a broad or global view of the world) specifies the definitions of the concepts or ideas of the metaparadigm. It is in the process of defining the universal concepts of the nursing metaparadigm that the development of a nursing philosophy occurs. Theories are then derived from these definitions. A researcher uses these concept definitions as a starting point to develop a particular theory. For example, the definitions of person, environment, health, and nursing that you just wrote are the groundwork of your nursing theory.

Researchers have developed their particular philosophies into conceptual models or frameworks that are referred to as **paradigms.** *Paradigm* is a term used to explain the existing network of science, philosophy, and theory accepted by the field of nursing. These conceptual models (established examples) serve as a guide to systematically test a proposed theory and to verify the theory's appropriateness for application to nursing practice. These frameworks are sometimes borrowed from other scientific fields, such as sociology or psychology, and applied to the field of nursing.

A **theory** is an abstract statement that explains the relationship of concepts. In essence, a theory is a set of organized information that explains facts, ideas, principles, or laws. With regard to nursing, theory is the organized body of information about phenomena that is unique to nursing. Nursing theories provide nursing with a set of guidelines that give nurses a real purpose, meaning, and value; a framework that will support what we do, how we do it, and when we do it. Nursing theories support measures to improve quality care by collecting scientific data. Figure 10–1 outlines the steps in theory development.

$\mathcal{S}$ CIENTIFIC THEORIES INFLUENCING NURSING THEORY

Science, philosophy, and theory are parts of any scientific discipline. As a science, nursing is considered to be a new field; in fact, there is little reference to the field of nursing as a science before the 1950s. Compared to other scientific fields as they relate to theory, nursing is in its infancy.

To develop its knowledge base as a science, nursing borrowed from established scientific fields such as psychology and sociology. An example of the use of knowledge from other fields to build nursing as a science is Abraham Maslow's Theory of Human Motivation and Hierarchy of Human Needs. Maslow's theoretical model contributed to nursing practice by determining the order of importance in which nurses address the needs of clients. Maslow proposed that human

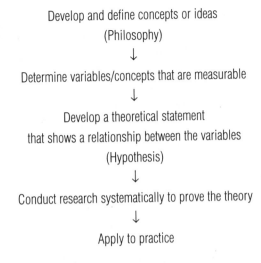

Develop and define concepts or ideas
(Philosophy)
↓
Determine variables/concepts that are measurable
↓
Develop a theoretical statement
that shows a relationship between the variables
(Hypothesis)
↓
Conduct research systematically to prove the theory
↓
Apply to practice

Figure 10–1 Steps in theory development.

motivation could be explained by five levels of human needs. The first level represents very basic needs such as food and water. The second level is the need for safety and security. The third level is the need for love and belonging. The fourth level is self-esteem, and the fifth is self-actualization (Frisch & Frisch, 2002). Maslow's theory for understanding human behavior is just one example of how nursing theory developed as a discipline using psychological and other scientific theories as a foundation. However, because nursing deals with the complexity of clients, nursing needed to develop its own body of science and scientific knowledge. In this instance, **science** is defined as the observation, identification, description, experimental investigation, and theoretical explanation of natural phenomena (Tomey & Alligood, 2002). Science gives meaning to who nurses are and what they do; that is, it defines the paradigm of nursing.

Nurses in the early era of nursing did not provide poor or unsafe care; they did what they thought was best based on values and thinking of their time. The continued development of a scientific base for nursing practice should be a high priority for the discipline. These are exciting times for the nursing profession as the foundation of knowledge continues to grow and expand. It is important to recognize the nursing leaders who have worked so hard over the last centuries to help develop this body of knowledge for nursing.

In the 1960s and 1970s nursing theorists began investigating issues pertaining to nursing. This theory development focused on the academic needs of nursing students. They developed appropriate curricula for each of the different levels of nursing. Then, in the mid-1970s, there was a change of focus and a new goal to make nursing more than a vocation but, rather, a profession (Tomey & Alligood, 2002). In the 1980s the universally accepted concepts of the nursing metaparadigm (person, environment, health, and nursing) were developed and lead to a more organized and consistent body of knowledge for nursing. Nursing theory was accepted in nursing and in nursing education programs (Tomey & Alligood). The acceptance of nursing theory allowed nursing leaders to begin publishing and presenting their newfound knowledge in journals, newspapers, books, and oral presentations. In the 1990s debates began as to whether nursing is a basic science, an applied science, or a practical science. Nursing's central concepts were defined in nursing literature. Scholars were trying to demonstrate the connection between nursing as an art and nursing as a science.

The "scientists" for the field of nursing are referred to as **nursing theorists.** Many of them have devoted a large part of their careers to theory development and should be commended and respected for their great efforts. Theorists have worked in a systematic manner. They have made the stages of theory development explicit so that others can review, replicate, and test a theory to give it **validity** (i.e., prove the theory's accuracy). The major theorists have worked hard to define nursing as a profession with their own body of knowledge. Each of these theorists has developed her theory based on her definitions of the metaparadigm of nursing. Refer to Table 10–2 for a list of a few of the nursing theorists who have worked to further the development of the field of nursing. There are many others who have contributed to the growth and development of nursing over the years. It is important for us as nurses to study these theorists and their theories in order to gain a better understanding of where nursing has been, where it is now, and where it will go. No one theory encompasses all of the ideas or concepts of nursing, and there may never be one, due to the complexity of dealing with human beings. Nursing theorists will continue to develop new theories to improve the practice of nursing.

Table 10-2 Nursing theorists' contribution to nursing

Theorist	Theory	Description of theory	Application to nursing
Florence Nightingale	Environmental Theory	A belief that a person's surroundings such as clean air, water, and lighting can play a part in their healing process and their quality of care.	Made nurses more aware of the environment in which the clients receive care.
Virginia Henderson	Definition of Nursing	Nurses should help a client regain as much independence as quickly as possible with a holistic approach.	Helps us treat each client as an individual, including them in the plan of care and assisting them with a quick and healthy recovery.
Jean Watson	Philosophy and Science of Caring	Supports the idea of humanistic and holistic care; focus is on "caring," promoting health, and preventing illness.	Focuses on the importance of the "caring" relationship and communication in an individual's health.
Patricia Benner	From Novice to Expert: Excellence and Power in Clinical Nursing Practice	Nurses move through stages of expertise and skill as they practice nursing; defines a set of competencies from novice to expert nurse.	Has made nursing aware of effects of clinical skills on client care and client outcomes. Benner's goal was to make the community more aware of nursing as a responsible and caring practice.
Dorothea Orem	Self-Care Deficit Theory of Nursing	Nurses assist clients to their highest level of self-care.	Has made nurses more of aware of individualized client care, their participation in plan of care and return to their highest possible level of self-care.

Table 10-2 (continued)

Theorist	Theory	Description of theory	Application to nursing
Martha Rogers	Unitary Human Beings	Human beings are the focus of nursing. Humans and their environments are made up of energy fields and are continually working together to maintain harmony.	Supports and encourages scientific research and professional development of nursing; encourages letting go of tradition and constantly building on continued education. Rogers continued to expand her knowledge base and theory ideas to keep current with technological advances.
Imogene King	Systems Framework and Theory of Goal Attainment	Involves three systems: personal, interpersonal, and social; these systems form the connection between the client and the nurse. These components make up the process of nursing.	Encourages nurses to collaborate with each client to determine individualized goals and their plan of care.
Betty Neuman	Systems Model	A wholistic approach to client care; addresses the homeostasis of the client and the environmental effects with a focus on primary prevention.	Nurses use this theory in the clinical area, classrooms, and in continued research to prevent illness and encourage health through a wholistic systems approach to assessment and client-centered care; includes the client at the center of care; encourages continued research and growth with nursing knowledge and theories.

Table 10–2 (continued)

Theorist	Theory	Description of theory	Application to nursing
Hildegard Peplau	Psychodynamic Nursing	Client-nurse relationships use interpersonal skills and knowledge gained through previous research from other disciplines; you must understand your own behavior before you can help someone else understand his behavior.	Used in the mental health field to develop therapeutic interpersonal communication skills in meeting the needs of each client.
Madeline Leininger	Culture Care: Diversity and Universality Theory	Culturally specific care is provided in a "caring" manner.	Encourages nurses to gain an awareness of the uniqueness of each culture to meet the individualized needs of each client.
Rosemarie Rizzo Parse	Human Becoming	Views nursing as a human science that can function independently; attention is focused on individual definitions of health and quality of life and assists in making the client and the nurse partners in the plan of care.	Allows nursing the opportunity to grow into a profession with its own body of knowledge and a special approach to each individual client.
Nola Pender	Health Promotion Model	Health promotion for all ages is the priority in nursing care.	Refocuses nurses on health promotion and disease prevention.

$\mathscr{N}$URSING THEORY AS A BASIS FOR PRACTICE

Nurses at all levels of education play a very important role in nursing theory and research today.

Now that we have explored nursing theory, you may be wondering how your role as a nurse with an associate degree is related to nursing theory. Nurses at all levels of education play a very important role in nursing theory and research today. The associate degree–prepared nurse assists with problem identification, assists with data collection, and utilizes research findings in practice to improve the quality of client care. The baccalaureate-prepared nurse also helps identify problems, collect data, use research findings in practice, and analyze research literature. The master's-prepared nurse collaborates in research projects, and the doctorate–prepared nurse conducts independent, funded research projects (see Table 10–3) (Burns & Grove, 2001). You have an important role in research and nursing theories as an associate degree prepared nurse. With the team approach to research the field of nursing will continue to grow as a science with a respected and specialized body of knowledge.

CRITICAL THINKING ACTIVITY

1. Review your nursing practice and think of a situation that could be researched to promote a change in client care. Write about this situation.

_____

_____

_____

$\mathscr{R}$ELATIONSHIP OF THEORY TO PRACTICE

Theory, practice, and research are related and intertwined. They all work together to demonstrate nursing as a science using nursing's body of knowledge to guide nursing practice. The application of nursing theory to nursing practice depends on the skills of observation, questioning, and comparing/contrasting what is observed (Johnson & Webber, 2001). It is nursing theory that guides the practice of nursing in an effective manner. Research tests the theories and questions

Table 10–3 Nursing roles in nursing theory

Nursing Role	Relationship to Nursing Theory
Associate Degree–Prepared Nurse	The ASN notices that her surgical clients have better outcomes and are discharged sooner when family has been allowed unlimited visitation and keeps a record of this.
Baccalaureate–Prepared Nurse	The BSN does a literature review and finds that the literature verifies the assumption that the emotional support surgical clients receive from their families contributes to better outcomes and shorter hospital stays. She applies this acquired knowledge to her nursing practice by encouraging family interactions with clients.
Master–Prepared Nurse	The MSN collaborates in a research project that seeks to prove that emotional support provided to surgical clients by their families contributes to better outcomes and shorter hospital stays.
Doctorate–Prepared Nurse	The Ph.D. RN conducts research funded by a health-related organization to determine if family support promotes better outcomes and/or reduces hospital stays for surgical clients.

that arise in nursing practice. Nursing practice applies theory and research in client care. Nursing practice provides the study questions for research that is relevant to the field of nursing. Theory, practice, and research are interdependent (Kearney, 2001).

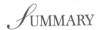 UMMARY

Nursing is a profession supported by scientific knowledge.

Nursing is a profession supported by scientific knowledge. As we practice nursing, we gain knowledge from our experiences that we can use to enlarge our scientific knowledge base. In other words, the art of nursing, or the care we provide, lends itself to the science of nursing. As nurses, we practice using principles provided by our metaparadigm and nursing theory. This principle-based practice provides us with the tools for critical thinking, client care, education, administration, research, and collaboration (Kearney, 2001).

As you continue to grow personally and professionally, remember the professional role you play in the field of nursing. Ideas that you gain from your care of one client could easily benefit many more clients. Nursing theory begins with a simple idea or concept that someone or a group of individuals begins to question and develop into a researchable concept or idea. These new concepts or ideas may develop into the next research project or theory.

ᴄHAPTER REFLECTIONS

1. How does nursing theory affect nursing as a profession?
2. Share an idea or theory of yours that could improve client care.
3. How could you apply nursing theory to your own nursing practice?

REFERENCES

Burns, N., & Grove, S. (2001). *The practice of nursing research: Conduct, critique, and utilization* (4th ed.). Philadelphia: W.B. Saunders Company.

Frisch. N., & Frisch, L. (2002). *Psychiatric mental health nursing* (2nd ed.). Clifton Park, NY: Thomson Delmar Learning.

Johnson, B., & Webber, P. (2001). *An introduction to theory and reasoning in nursing.* Philadelphia: Lippincott.

Kearney, R. (2001). *Advancing your career: Concepts of professional nursing.* Philadelphia: F.A. Davis Company.

Tomey, A., & Alligood, M. (2002). *Nursing theorists and their work* (5th ed.). St. Louis, MO: Mosby.

SUGGESTED RESOURCES

Malinowski, A., & Stamler, L. (2001). Comfort: Exploration of the concept in nursing. *Journal of Advanced Nursing, (39)*6, 599–606.

Schwartz-Barcott, D., Patterson, B., Lusardi, P., & Farmer, B. (2002). From practice to theory: Tightening the link via three fieldwork strategies. *Journal of Advanced Nursing, (39)*3, 281–289.

Smith, C., Pace, K., Kochinda, C., Klein Beck, S., Koehler, J., & Popkess-Vawter, S. (2002). Caregiving effectiveness model evolution to a midrange theory of home care: A process for critique and replication. *Advances in Nursing Science, (25)*1, 50–64.

$\mathscr{C}$hapter 11
Ethical and Legal Considerations

▼ ▼ ▼ ▼ ▼ ▼ ▼

$\mathscr{L}$EARNING OBJECTIVES

By the end of this chapter, you should be able to:

1. List the organizations that regulate nursing practice.
2. Explain legal issues that affect nursing practice.
3. Define personal values.
4. Explain the relationship between ethical principles and nursing practice.
5. Explain an ethical decision-making process.

$\mathscr{K}$EY TERMS

Assault

Autonomy

Battery

Beneficence

Bioethics

Clinical ethics

Code of ethics

Confidentiality

Delegation

Deontology

Ethical rights

Ethics

HIPAA

Justice

Licensure

Malpractice

Mandatory licensure

Morals

Negligence

Nonbeneficence

Option rights

Protected health information

Rights

Standard of care

Utilitarianism

Values

Veracity

Welfare rights

*S*CENARIO

Paula, a new RN on a medical-surgical floor, often follows Deb, a nurse who has worked on the floor for many years. Several times clients have complained that they have asked for pain medication and not received it. When Paula has reviewed the medication records on these clients, she notes that Deb has charted that each client received pain medication at each prn interval that was ordered. Paula notices that sometimes when Deb gives her report she is somewhat disoriented. Paula is not certain what is happening, and she also feels that she is new and could be rocking the boat if she says anything about her concerns.

*T*HINK ABOUT IT

1. Have you ever experienced an ethical situation that placed you in an awkward position?
2. Do you feel that it is your professional responsibility to report all ethical concerns?
3. Do you already feel that Deb is guilty of stealing client pain medications, or can you come up with alternative explanations?

$\mathcal{I}$NTRODUCTION

As nurses, we make numerous decisions about client care daily. This is an awesome responsibility! These decisions become more difficult when a variety of personal values and beliefs are involved. Conflict may occur between our values as the health care provider and the client's values and requests. At that point, moral and ethical decision making becomes a very important and valuable tool for a nurse. Ethical decisions may involve legal issues. The RN functions as a leader and is a vital member of the team involved in making ethical and legal decisions.

In this chapter we will review key ethical and legal principles that will be important for you to understand as you transition into your new RN role. We will discuss the development of personal values and their influence on ethical issues and the ethical decision-making process. We will explore how nursing practice is guided by legislative acts and client rights. An ethical decision-making process will be presented to guide nurses in making ethical decisions. Finally, we will discuss how values, ethics, legal issues, and ethical decision making influence nurses and the nursing care they provide.

$\mathcal{V}$ALUES AND ETHICS

Values are beliefs that guide our thoughts and actions.

Why do we make the decisions we make? How do we decide the appropriate actions in various situations? Personal values and beliefs drive our decisions. **Values** are beliefs that guide our thoughts and actions. We develop these values from our family, friends, culture, and environment. In a sense, our values are our philosophy of life.

Our values determine our ethics or our code of conduct. We form professional values and ethics from our personal backgrounds and educational systems. Professional values and ethics determine our thoughts and response in ethical dilemmas that we face with clients.

Morals, Ethics, and Bioethics

Morals are the rules of right and wrong that serve as the standard for decision making and behavior.

Morals, ethics, and *bioethics* are key terms to understanding the principles of ethics. **Morals** are the rules of right and wrong that serve as the standard for decision making and behavior. An example of a moral is "Good people do not cheat." Therefore, desiring to be an upright citizen, one does not cheat.

Lawrence Kohlberg (1977) studied the development of morals in individuals. Kohlberg was not concerned with the morality of a decision but concentrated on the reasons people make decisions. He described three levels and six stages of moral development from childhood to adulthood (see Table 11–1). The first level is called the preconventional, or premoral, level. In this level, a child makes decisions based on fear of the consequences of actions rather than respect for the authority figure. The second level is the conventional level. The individual makes decisions based on a desire to conform to the norms of the family, group, community, or nation. The third level is the postconventional, or principled, level. The individual is not concerned with conforming to the group but, rather, makes decisions based on an internalized set of rules (Kozier, Erb, Berman, & Snyder, 2004).

Ethics define how people should act because of the moral standard. An ethicist is concerned about the morality of a decision and would analyze the moral standard to see if it is correct in all circumstances. Ethics involve the analysis of actions. For example, an ethicist would analyze whether cheating is appropriate in some circumstances. **Bioethics** (also known as **clinical ethics**) applies ethical theories and principles to health care situations.

Code of Ethics

A code of ethics is the standard that members of a profession follow when performing the duties of the profession.

A **code of ethics** is the standard that members of a profession follow when performing the duties of the profession. The nursing code of ethics is the standard that nurses should follow when providing nursing care. As members of the community see members of the nursing profession following the standard, or code of ethics, community members will view

Table 11–1 Piaget's cognitive stages and Kohlberg's stages of development of moral judgment

Piaget's Cognitive Stages	Kohlberg's Stages of Development of Moral Judgment
Sensorimotor (birth to 2 years): begins to acquire language	
Task: Object permanence	
Sensorimotor continues	Preconventional Level:
Preoperational (2 to 7 years) begins: use of representational thought	1. Morality Stage: Avoid punishment by not breaking rules of authority figures
Task: Use language and mental images to think and communicate	
Preoperational continues	2. Individualism, Instrumental Purpose, and Exchange Stage: "Right" is relative, follow rules when in own interest
	Conventional Level:
Preoperational continues	3. Mutual Expectations, Relationships, and Conformity to Moral Norms Stage: Need to be "good" in own and others' eyes, believe in rules and regulations
Concrete Operations (7 to 12 years)	
begins: engage in inductive reasoning and concrete problem solving	
Task: Learn concepts of conservation and reversibility	
Formal Operations (12 years to adulthood):	4. Social System and Conscience Stage:
engage in abstract reasoning and analytical problem solving	Uphold laws because they are fixed social duties
Task: Develop a workable philosophy of life	
Formal Operations continues	Postconventional Level:
	5. Social Contract or Utility and Individual Rights Stage: Uphold laws in the interest of the greatest good for the greatest number; uphold laws that protect universal rights
	6. Universal Ethical Principles Stage: Support universal moral principles regardless of the price for doing so

(From *Health Assessment and Physical Examination,* 2nd ed., by M. Estes, 2002, Clifton Park, NY: Thomson Delmar Learning.)

the members of the profession as reliable, trustworthy, and accountable. The American Nurses Association has established the code of ethics for nurses. The International Council of Nurses also has developed a code of ethics for nursing, the ICN Code of Ethics. Refer to appendixes E and F. The National Student Nurses' Association provides a code of ethics for you to follow as a student nurse. It can be found at www.nsna.org. It sets the standards for professional conduct and academic and clinical conduct, introducing students to the ideals and principles of the nursing profession. These become an important component in the holistic and professional development of the new RN.

Ethical Theories

An ethical theory is a framework for personal beliefs that guide one's values, decisions, and actions and determines responses in life.

Why do I make the decisions I make? What guides my actions? What determines how I respond to my neighbor? An ethical theory is a framework for personal beliefs that guide one's values, decisions, and actions and determines responses in life. Therefore, it is important for us to study the foundation of ethical theories to determine how an individual will make decisions and respond in life.

One of those theories is **utilitarianism** (or situational ethics). It was first proposed by David Hume (1711–1776) and further developed by Jeremy Bentham (1748–1826) and John Stuart Mill (1806–1873). The two supporting concepts of utilitarianism are:

1. "Achieve the greatest good for the greatest number." In other words, "utilitarian values give greater moral weight to the needs of the many than to the needs of the few, even if the few are much worse off." (Hein, 2001, p. 245)
2. "The ends justify the means."

According to this theory, an individual does not have rights but is considered as one with the whole population. The right action would be the action by which the greatest number of people would benefit. The situation determines whether an action is done with honor or is morally right or wrong.

An example of utilitarianism is spending more federal money on people with curable diseases than on the smaller number of people with incurable diseases. In the movie *Pearl Harbor,* casualties were so numerous that the hospital personnel and facility could not care for all the injured. A nurse was asked to assess all incoming clients to determine which ones could be assisted and which ones were too badly injured to benefit from assistance. This is an example of triage, an accepted concept in health care.

A second example of a theory is from Immanuel Kant (1724–1804), who developed the theory of **deontology.** This theory states that the right or wrong of an action is dependent upon the morality of the action. The action is moral if it is based on good will. To do one's duty is right or good, not to do one's duty is wrong. This theory is further divided into two ideologies: *act deontology* and *rule deontology.*

Act deontology gathers all the facts about a situation and determines the appropriate action. The generalized decision then becomes the right action or judgment for all similar situations. These rules regarding actions or judgments then apply to all similar situations, even if the external circumstances surrounding the situation change.

Rule deontology states that principles or rules determine our actions. These principles or rules do not change with the situation. A rule could be "Never cheat another person" or "Always be kind to elderly people." This rule applies in all situations. Rule deontologists are not concerned with consequences or the situations in which the rule is applied, only that the rule is followed. A nursing example of rule deontology is the rule in most facilities that states, "Clients must be turned every two hours." If the rule is followed, the client is turned every two hours regardless of her desires or condition. What if the client is terminally ill and in severe pain? What if the client refuses to be turned? Is the rule still followed?

Ethical Principles

Ethical principles are based on the right of each person to be treated with respect (Chitty, 1997). Ethical principles are justice, autonomy, beneficence, and veracity.

Justice
Autonomy
Beneficence/nonbeneficence
Veracity

Box 11–1 Ethical principles affecting nursing

Justice

The principle of **justice** states that all people are to be treated fairly (Kearney, 2001). In nursing, this would indicate that all clients would receive quality care regardless of diagnosis, care needs, or financial concerns. This becomes a concern in the allocation of funds. Does the 89-year-old client with a terminal disease and multiple complications or the 20-year-old with a broken leg receive the funded care? Some would say that the 20-year-old should be given the care because the elderly man is going to die anyway. From this perspective, clients with terminal or extensive needs will not get the funds because others with lesser needs can be given more reasonable or equitable care. The principle of justice makes us question the ethics of a situation but does not provide the answers.

Autonomy

Autonomy is based on self-determination and independence. Autonomy provides each person the option to make personal decisions and act on those decisions. Thus, each person has the right to determine her personal health care (Chitty, 1997; Kearney, 2001). Health care workers following the principle of autonomy respect each individual person to make sound decisions. Strictly taken, autonomy offers the individual the right to make a health care decision, even if the nursing staff does not agree. An example is an 18-year-old client who is a Jehovah's Witness and is refusing a needed blood transfusion. In this case, the client has the right to refuse the blood transfusion even if the nurses caring for her disagree with her decision. However, if the same client had tuberculosis or a highly contagious disease that could harm others, she could be isolated for the good of society. Thus a client's autonomy can sometimes be overruled.

A nurse is not allowed to withhold information from a client to prevent her from making a decision with which she disagrees. She must inform the client of all health care options and provide care even if the client's health care decision differs from the nurse's beliefs.

Beneficence/Nonbeneficence

A nurse's duty is to do good or promote the well-being of clients **(beneficence)** and not to intentionally or unintentionally harm the client **(nonbeneficence)** (Rosenthal, 2001). Good care requires not only technical skill but also having a holistic view of the client that includes the client's values, beliefs, feelings, and desires. The nurse providing good care also considers the family's and significant other's input. A problem arises if the nurse does not agree with what the client thinks is good care. Who then can make the best ethical decision about the client's care? The nurse can discuss the situation with colleagues and physicians involved in the case. If she still has concerns after discussing the situation with others involved in the case, sometimes the situation can be referred to an ethical committee within the facility.

Nonbeneficence also has another aspect that requires the nurse to protect from harm those who cannot care for themselves, such as the mentally challenged, the elderly, or children. The nurse guards the best interests of these clients and seeks quality, equitable care. For example, the nurse reports possible abuse or neglect cases.

Veracity

Veracity is the principle of truthfulness. Nurses have a responsibility to be truthful with clients. Trust is the basis of an open, sincere, meaningful relationship, and the basis of trust is truthfulness. Health care workers have a responsibility to share truthful information with their clients. It is difficult to share bad news with clients. We could rationalize that the client is better off not knowing everything, or that she would not understand the information. These are not legitimate reasons to withhold truthful information from a client. Even if a client withholds truthful information from the health care worker, such as facts about her sex life, a socially unacceptable disease, or mental illness, the nurse does not have the right to withhold information from the client.

The Client's Rights

A right is something a person can lay claim to or an entitlement that seems due a person.

The principles discussed in the preceding text are based on **rights.** Ellis and Hartley (2004) define a right as "something that is owed to an individual on a legal, moral, or ethical basis" (p. 316). A right is something a person can lay claim to or an entitlement that seems due a person. Rights may also be described as a person's privileges, special considerations, or freedoms. There are three rights: *welfare rights* (legal rights), *ethical rights* (moral rights), and *option rights* (Aiken, 2004).

Welfare rights (legal rights) are a legal access or right to something that will give an individual an advantage or gain. In the United States everyone has a right to employment regardless of race, religion, or gender. Laws protect these rights. If an individual's rights are violated, she may appeal to a legal system for justice.

Ethical rights (moral rights) are based on a moral or ethical principle. Law does not support these rights. However, over time the belief in these principles gives them the conceptual backing of a legal right. An example of this is health care in the United States. Many people believe that everyone has the right to receive health care, but obtaining appropriate health care is not a legal right.

Option rights are based on the dignity and freedom of choice of all individuals. As U.S. citizens, we have the freedom to choose where we live, the type of clothes we wear, and, in most cases, where we travel. This is because our country believes in the right of each individual to make choices and to have the free will to follow those choices as long as they do not infringe on the rights of others.

Summary of Ethical Principles

Concerns arise from ethical principles and the interpretation of individual rights. "When a conflict of rights arises, how should the conflict be resolved? Obligations to clients may seem to conflict with obligations to the physician or to the institution. This is not really a moral dilemma although the decision may be an agonizing one. An important distinction is made between doing what is morally right and what is least difficult practically" (Hood & Leddy, 2003). Do we take the action that is morally right, or the action that is least difficult? Which can be more agonizing? Doing what is morally right? Or taking the road of least resistance and then living with your conscience regarding the results of the actions? Ethical decision making is discussed in the next section.

CRITICAL THINKING ACTIVITIES

1. List some of your personal values.

   _____

   _____

   _____

2. Write your philosophy of nursing.

   _____

   _____

   _____

3. Review the American Nurses Association Code of Ethics (Appendix E) and discuss it in class. Jot down some ideas you would like to discuss.

   _____

   _____

   _____

4. Ethical Principle Scenario:

   Deana, a 76-year-old woman, has Parkinson's disease. She had an athletic build and has been very active her entire life. Slowly, the effects of Parkinson's have overtaken her body. Because her family is unable to care for her any longer in the home, she has been admitted to a nursing home. She is unable to walk and needs to be lifted from a wheelchair to her bed. Recently a swallow test was done indicating that she is unable to swallow any type of food. She is losing weight and a small pressure sore is developing on her coccyx. She has had aspiration pneumonia twice in the last three months. The nursing home director has requested permission from the family for placement of a feeding tube. The family refuses to have any type of feeding tube inserted, knowing that she will starve to death.

Refer back to the preceding discussion of ethical concepts. Put yourself in the place of the client, the client's family, and the nursing home personnel in the scenario for this Critical Thinking Activity. What would be your viewpoint as the client, the client's family, and nursing home personnel based on the ethical principles of justice, autonomy, beneficence, nonbeneficence, veracity, and client's rights? Refer to the example that is given here in the justice section and then write your own thoughts for the other five principles. Discuss your thoughts with your peers.

Evaluate the scenario from the viewpoint of the client, the client's family, and nursing home personnel as their views may relate to the ethical principle of justice.

Ethical principle	Ethical principle as it relates to the client, the client's family, and nursing home personnel
Justice	Client:
	My body has deteriorated and I would like a natural, dignified death.
	Family:
	We have provided the best care we can. The family's funds have been depleted in providing nursing home care. We feel she has suffered enough and prolonging life will only cause more suffering.
	Nursing home personnel:
	The nursing home director has offered nutritional supplements to provide quality nutritional care. Some of the nursing home personnel do not think Deana is being treated fairly because the family is starving her to death.
Autonomy	Client:
	Family:
	Nursing home personnel:

Beneficence   Client:

Family:

Nursing home personnel:

Nonbeneficence   Client:

Family:

Nursing home personnel:

Veracity   Client:

Family:

Nursing home personnel:

Client's rights   Client:

Family:

Nursing home personnel:

$\mathcal{E}$THICAL DECISION MAKING

To make an ethical decision, a nurse needs to review ethical principles, evaluate personal values and beliefs, and research related legal issues.

Earlier in this book, we discussed how the nursing process is the basis for decision making in nursing. Now we will see how the steps of the nursing process relate to the ethical decision–making process.

Nurses face many ethical issues. To make an ethical decision, a nurse needs to review ethical principles, evaluate personal values and beliefs, and research related legal issues. Chitty (1997) presented an ethical decision–making process with the following six steps:

1. **Clarifying the ethical dilemma**—What is the ethical problem? Who owns the problem? Who will be affected by the problem and results of the problem? What ethical principles are related to the problem? Is there a conflict with personal and professional values or professional duties? What is the time frame for making the decision?

2. **Gathering data**—How did this situation occur? Have all parties been contacted and had input into the situation? Has a legal and ethical literature review been completed? Are there any political or economic issues to consider?

3. **Identifying options**—Brainstorm and list all possible solution options. List new and creative alternatives.

4. **Making a decision**—Consider the pros and cons of the outcome of each potential solution. Consider ethical ramifications of each solution. Will other dilemmas occur because of the potential decision? Will any institutional, community, or government policies be affected? Make a decision. Not making a decision is not being accountable or responsible.

5. **Choosing a course of action**—Outline a plan of action to carry out the decision. Make sure that personal values and morals are not compromised. Communicate appropriately with all involved parties. Act as a team when completing the course of action.

6. **Evaluating the decision**—Analyze all the unexpected outcomes produced by the ethical dilemma. It is not uncommon that a decision made regarding a crisis ethical situation may result in

other unsettled issues. Review and address all issues that arise. Only after a decision is made and the results of the decision occur can it be determined if it was the best decision. Evaluate if the best decision was made. If an alternative decision had been made, what would be the results? Are there any legal implications that need addressing? Are new policies needed or do other policies need changing because of the chosen decision and actions?

The steps in the ethical decision–making process have many parallels to the nursing process (see Table 11–2).

Table 11–2 Comparison of the nursing process and the ethical decision-making process

Ethical Decision-Making Process	Nursing Process
Clarify the ethical dilemma.	Assess patient needs.
Gather data.	Decide on appropriate nursing diagnosis.
Identify options.	Plan nursing care.
Make a decision.	
Choose a course of action.	Implement nursing action.
Evaluate the decision.	Evaluate outcomes.

CRITICAL THINKING ACTIVITY

1. Using the ethical decision–making process presented in this chapter, discuss with your peers the best approach in handling Paula's situation in the chapter's opening scenario. Write your decisions for each section in the following chart.

Ethical decision–making step	Student's thoughts
Clarifying the ethical dilemma	
Gathering data	
Identifying options	
Making a decision	
Choosing a course of action	
Evaluating the decision	

$\mathcal{R}$EGULATION OF NURSING PRACTICE

A license is a legal document issued by each state to certify that a person has met minimum standards to qualify as a practitioner.

Licensure is mandatory for a nurse to practice nursing. A license is a legal document issued by each state to certify that a person has met minimum standards to qualify as a practitioner. Each state is responsible to its citizens to provide qualified, competent health care personnel. Each state has a nurse practice act that defines the requirements for licensure as an RN.

All 50 states use the National Council Licensure Examination for Registered Nurses (NCLEX-RN) to license nurses. To be eligible to take the examination, a student must graduate from a state-approved school of nursing and be approved by the State Board of Nursing. The NCLEX-RN is a computerized test given to nursing graduates at a local testing site. The candidate for licensure must pass the exam to be licensed and registered in the state. A nurse licensed in one state may apply for licensure in another state. The license is permanent but must be renewed periodically by paying a fee to the state where licensure is desired.

All states require **mandatory licensure** of nurses, meaning that a nurse must have a license to practice legally in that state. All states license and register graduates of all nursing education programs.

$\mathcal{L}$EGAL ISSUES

Nurses are accountable for their own actions. Even though states regulate nursing practice by licensure and the state's nurse practice act, nurses are vulnerable to several types of legal action. Some legal concepts that the nurse should understand are: torts, negligence, malpractice, delegation, assault and battery, informed consent, and confidentiality.

> Torts
> Negligence
> Malpractice
> Delegation
> Assault and battery
> Informed consent
> Confidentiality

Box 11–2 Legal issues affecting nurses

Torts

Torts may be an intentional or unintentional civil wrong against a person that results in physical, emotional, or economic harm. An intentional act is a willful act against another person's rights or property; however, a tort needs no proof of intent to cause harm. An example of a tort is a nurse's accidentally using the wrong solution to irrigate a client's bladder.

Negligence

Negligence is committing an act that a reasonable, prudent person would not have done in the same or similar situation or failing to act as a reasonable, prudent person would have acted in the same or similar situation. For an act to be negligent, it does not need proof of premeditation or intent to harm, but it does require that proof of specific damage or harm was done. An example of negligence is a person's driving on a narrow road, seeing a bicycler, and not slowing down. The driver hits the bicycler and causes injury to her.

Malpractice

Malpractice is professional negligence. Malpractice occurs when a professional person does not act as another reasonable, prudent professional person would have acted in the same or similar situation because of a lack of "professional knowledge, experience, or skill that can be expected of others in the profession" (Como, 2002, p. 1047). This action is classified as an unintentional tort because there is no need to prove that the professional intended to cause harm or be negligent. Malpractice includes acts of commission and acts of omission. An act of commission is committing an act that should not be done. An act of omission is not doing an act that should have been done. Acts of commission and acts of omission are grounds for legal action. In legal action, evidence must be presented that the nurse did not meet the standard of care. The **standard of care** is the minimal requirement of competent care that does not harm a client. The nursing standard of care is what a reasonable, prudent nurse would do under the same or a similar situation.

"The prerequisite for a malpractice action is that the defendant (nurse) has specialized knowledge and skills and through the practice of that specialized knowledge caused the plaintiff's (patient's) injury" (Chitty, 1997, p. 514). There are several issues that need to occur for an act to be defined as malpractice: (1) a nurse assumes the duty of care or responsibility for the care of a client, (2) the nurse fails to meet the standard of care when caring for the client, (3) the client is injured because of the break in the standard of care, and (4) the injury is confirmed (Chitty). An example of negligence is a nurse's gossiping with co-workers and failing to answer a client's call light. Her failure to act resulted in the client's falling and breaking a hip when trying to go to the bathroom alone. Because of the nurse's actions or failure to act (negligence), the client was injured.

Not only is the nurse responsible for personal actions, but the facility is also legally responsible because of the legal *respondeat superior* (master-servant) rule. This rule states that the master is responsible for the actions of the servants. It implies that the nurse's employer or facility is responsible for the actions of the nurse.

Legal Implications of Nursing

There are several actions a nurse may take throughout the course of a day that may make her vulnerable to legal action. A review of some of these legal issues follows.

Delegation

Professional nurses have the authority to delegate nursing activities to other health care personnel.

Delegation is giving the authority for one person to act in the place of another. Professional nurses have the authority to delegate nursing activities to other health care personnel. The state nursing practice acts do not give LPNs/LVNs the right to delegate (Chitty, 1997). The professional nurse must know the scope of practice for the members of the health care team and delegate accordingly. She is held accountable for the actions of the persons to whom she delegates. The health care personnel are responsible for safely performing the delegated activity. Because the main concern in delegation is the safety of the client, the professional nurse needs to assess the capabilities of the person to whom the activity is delegated to make sure it will be completed safely. A nurse is responsible to refuse an action that is not within her scope of practice or expertise, regardless of who requests her to perform the act.

Assault and Battery

Assault is a threat or an attempt to make physical contact with a person who does not desire the contact. **Battery** is a completed assault whereby a person has had physical contact with another person without her consent or permission. An example of a potential battery is giving a client an injection without proper consent, or performing surgery on an unconscious client without consent.

Informed Consent

An informed consent requires that a competent client be given accurate and full information to make a prudent, knowledgeable, voluntary decision to consent to treatment.

An informed consent prevents an assault by having a client give written consent for treatment. An informed consent requires that a competent client be given accurate and full information to make a prudent, knowledgeable, voluntary decision to consent to treatment (Rosenthal, 2001). To be "competent" indicates that the client has the mental capacity to comprehend the information given about the procedure or treatment. A knowledgeable decision is based on the completeness of provided information. Voluntary consent implies freedom to make the choice without "undue influences" (Rosenthal, p. 4). Information given to a client should include risks, benefits, side effects, costs, and other options.

Confidentiality

HIPAA ensures that the right people use the client's information appropriately and discreetly for the right purposes.

Confidentiality is the safe handling of client information or the ability to keep a secret. Confidentiality is not a new concept at all, but, rather, an old concept with new standards and disciplinary actions attached as consequences for those who choose not to comply with new regulations. Nurses have access to private information about clients. It is the nurse's responsibility to protect the client's private health care information. This does not mean that the nurse cannot share needed information with the appropriate people, such as the doctor or other health care personnel. It does mean that the nurse must make a conscientious effort to share it only with the appropriate people and to involve the client in this decision process.

In 1996 the Health Insurance Portability and Accountability Act **(HIPAA)** was enacted to ensure health care coverage for employees when they were changing jobs. The act soon grew into multiple regulations for the health care system. Technology boomed and offered an array of advances for the health care environment including electronic medical records. Confidentiality became an even greater concern in health care. It is important that the client be protected and that there be no misuse of personal health information. All health care facilities were required to comply with the new HIPAA Privacy Regulations by April 14, 2003 ("HIPAA Privacy Policies").

Health care personnel do not have an option in following the HIPAA guidelines. The guidelines are mandatory for everyone. HIPAA protects the client from unauthorized personnel's gaining access to private health information. HIPAA ensures that the right people use the client's information appropriately and discreetly for the right purposes.

HIPAA Privacy Regulations require a facility to give the client a copy of the facility's written Notice of Privacy Practices when an individual enters any health care facility for treatment. The Notice of Privacy Practices informs the client of ways the facility plans to access, use, and disclose the client's protected health information. The client is required to sign a statement indicating that she received the information. If the client does not sign the statement of receipt of HIPAA information, health care personnel are required to document that the client did not sign the notice and the reason for not signing the notice. Facility personnel are required to offer the client an opportunity to ask questions regarding the notice. The facility is required to keep the written statement of notice receipt on record for at least six years.

HIPAA requires that any information that could be used to trace a client's identity or lead to access of the client's medical information be protected. This information is referred to as **protected health information (PHI).** Information about the client's past, present, or future physical or psychological condition also falls under protected health information.

Information that can be disclosed without the client's consent is information shared between two doctors providing treatment to the client, between nurses directly providing care to the client, or between billing personnel to receive payment for the services provided. Before any protected health information can be disclosed to a third party, the client must give written authorization for the disclosure except for reasons related to treatment, payment, or health care operations.

Health care personnel have a responsibility to protect client privacy. If HIPAA regulations are not followed, the health care personnel are liable to receive disciplinary actions. The Department of Health and Human Services' Office for Civil Rights (OCR) enforces civil disciplinary actions for violations of the HIPAA Privacy Regulations. The Department of Justice prosecutes criminal issues (www.hhs.gov/news/press/2002pres). The new standards and regulations developed through

HIPAA are meant to empower clients and directly involve them in decisions regarding their medical records. The regulations force health care personnel to always be aware and to respect their clients' rights.

One example that might help explain the seriousness of this issue is that individuals previously may have been hesitant to get lab tests done for fear that the test results could be accessed without their knowledge or consent. For example, a person having tests done to detect the presence of cancer genes or HIV might have had some serious concerns about confidentiality with insurance companies and employers. If the person applied for insurance but the potential insurance company obtained the test results, the company might have refused coverage. A potential employer having access to test results might have refused employment to the job applicant. This situation actually occurred in the 1970s, when some African Americans who tested positive for sickle-cell anemia were denied jobs by major airlines and were required to pay higher prices for health insurance coverage (Rosenthal, 2001). Situations of this type brought about confidentiality reform in legislative acts.

CRITICAL THINKING ACTIVITY

1. Review your state's Nurse Practice Act. Nurse Practice Acts for each state can be accessed at the state's board of nursing Web site. Identify five items that you learned or rethought as you read your state's Nurse Practice Act. Share these thoughts with your peers.

   _____
   _____
   _____
   _____
   _____

POTENTIAL FUTURE ETHICAL CONCERNS

We have discussed ethical situations that nurses face such as tube feeding usage, reporting potential drug abuse by health care personnel, allocation of funds in client care, appropriate administration of blood, reporting neglect and abuse cases, and confidentiality of the client's private health care information. Some potential future ethical issues are gene research, cloning, and allocation of funds for the elderly versus younger, healthier people. As health care systems move in more of a profit-oriented direction, nurses may feel pulled between issues of nursing practice and economic shortcuts. These are only a few of the ethical situations you as nurses will face in coming years. As you transition into the role of an RN, it is important that you examine the origin and development of your personal values and make the determination to provide quality care to your clients within those preset value parameters.

In your new role as RN, you will face many ethical and legal situations and be expected to function professionally as a leader and decision maker.

SUMMARY

Nurses face many situations every day that could become legal or ethical issues. Personal values influence our thoughts, opinions, and actions. Because a nurse is responsible for her personal actions, it is important that the nurse make wise decisions when caring for clients. By recalling ethical principles and legal nursing implications and following the ethical decision–making process, you will learn to make prudent decisions followed by prudent actions. In your new role as RN, you will face many ethical and legal situations and be expected to function professionally as a leader and decision maker. Determine your own values, beliefs, ethics, and moral ideas or opinions so that when you find yourself in such situations you are better equipped and ready to face the situation. Remember the importance of providing your clients with the best care possible.

CHAPTER REFLECTIONS

1. If you were Paula, would you approach Deb regarding the pain medication discrepancies?

2. Is approaching Deb the first step Paula should take? Why or why not?

3. What would be the ethical and legal implications to Deb if Paula went over Deb's head and was wrong?

4. How do your personal values and beliefs affect the way you would approach this situation?

REFERENCES

Aiken, T. (2004). *Legal, ethical, and political issues in nursing* (2nd ed.). Philadelphia: F.A. Davis Company.

Chitty, K. (1997). *Professional nursing: Concepts and challenge* (2nd ed.). Philadelphia: W.B. Saunders Company.

Como, D. (2002). *Mosby's medical, nursing, and allied health dictionary* (6th ed.). St. Louis, MO: Mosby.

Ellis, J., & Hartley, C. (2004). *Nursing in today's world: Trends, issues, and management* (8th ed.). Philadelphia: Lippincott Williams & Wilkins.

Kearney, R. (2001). *Advancing your career: Concepts of professional nursing.* Philadelphia: F.A. Davis Company.

Kohlberg, L. (1977). *Recent research in moral development.* New York: Holt, Rinehart, & Winston.

Kozier, B., Erb, G., Berman, A., & Snyder, S. (2004). *Fundamentals of nursing: Concepts, process, and practice* (7th ed.). Upper Saddle River, NJ: Prentice Hall.

Hein, E. (2001). *Nursing issues in the 21st century: Perspectives from the literature.* Philadelphia: Lippincott Williams & Wilkins.

HIPAA privacy policies core training module self-study version. http://www.healthlinkinc.com

Hood, L., & Leddy, S. (2003). *Leddy and Pepper's conceptual bases of professional nursing* (5th ed.). Philadelphia: Lippincott Williams & Wilkins.

Rosenthal, M. (2001). *Bioethics: What is the "right thing" in healthcare?* [On-line]. Available: http://www.sarahealth.com

SUGGESTED RESOURCES

Habel, M. (2003). *Bioethics: Strengthening nursing's role* [On-line]. Available: http://www.nurseweek.com

Ludwick, R., & Silva, M. (2000). *Nursing around the world: Cultural values and ethical conflicts* [On-line]. Available: http://www.nursingworld.org

National Student Nurses' Association. [On-line]. Available: http://www.nsna.org

U.S. Department of Justice. http://www.hhs.gov/news/press/2002pres

◢ppendix A
New NCLEX Question Format

▼ ▼ ▼ ▼ ▼ ▼ ▼

You have successfully taken the National Council Licensure Examination for Practical Nurses (NCLEX-PN). After you graduate from the RN program you will need to take the National Council Licensure Examination for Registered Nurses (NCLEX-RN) to legally practice as a licensed RN. The RN program equips you with knowledge and critical thinking skills for success on the NCLEX. It is important that you value your education experience and diligently apply yourself by reading your textbooks, attending class, utilizing learning opportunities in the clinical experiences, improving critical thinking skills, and interacting frequently with the program's faculty members.

The purpose of the NCLEX is to assess the entry-level competence of nursing candidates. The National Council of State Boards of Nursing (NCSBN) updates the NCLEX continually to keep the testing content current and consistent with new technological possibilities and advances. For example, in 1994 the NCSBN introduced computerized testing in place of the previous paper-and-pencil exam. On April 1, 2003, the NCSBN (2003) changed the question format on the NCLEX-RN to include alternate item response questions. The current NCLEX testing format of cognitive ability levels (knowledge, comprehension, application, and analysis) and its question content, consisting of the four major categories of client needs (safe, effective care environment; health promotion and maintenance; psychosocial integrity; and physiological integrity), as discussed in Chapter 3, are the same.

By adding the alternate item response questions, the exam utilizes opportunities provided by technology to assess candidate ability other than the standard multiple-choice questions. The NCLEX is now able to incorporate charts, tables, and graphic images into the test questions. Some of the alternate item response questions will require the candidate to complete math equations to correctly calculate an answer. These new alternate item response questions will be added to the standard multiple-choice questions on the NCLEX. The alternate item response questions have only been added to the NCLEX-RN to date, but they will be added to the NCLEX-PN in the next few years.

Three types of alternate item response questions that have been added to the NCLEX are the multiple-response multiple-choice question, the fill-in-the-blank question, and the identify-the-area question. You probably have taken exams with all of these types of questions at some time in the course of your education, but you may not be familiar with the terminology used for the question types. We will discuss each of these question types and give you a few sample questions. In the question example section, questions covering similar content are given for each type of alternate question so that you can see how the responses can vary.

You are familiar with the traditional multiple-choice question that typically has four answer choices from which you choose the *best* answer. In multiple-response multiple-choice questions, there are more than one correct answer and more than four choices. Rather than the question's including the phrase "choose the best answer," this type of question will include a phrase telling you to choose "at least two answers." You must choose all of the correct answers to be counted correct. Remember, when scoring the NCLEX, *no partial credit* is given for multiple-response multiple-choice questions. You must mark all the correct responses or you will get no credit.

Let's practice answering some multiple-response multiple-choice questions. Remember, there are *more than two correct answers* to each of the questions.

1. The cardiac landmarks, or the sites on the chest where the heart sounds are best heard, are the:
   Choose all that apply.
   ___ Aortic area
   ___ Erb's point
   ___ Bachmann's bundle
   ___ Costochondral junction
   ___ Pulmonic area
   ___ Xiphoid process
   Answer: aortic area, Erb's point, and pulmonic area

2. When listening for bowel sounds the nurse assesses four sections of the abdomen. These areas are called the:
Choose all that apply.

__ Right upper quadrant
__ Periumbilical region
__ Epigastric region
__ Left lower quadrant
__ Left upper quadrant

Answer: right upper quadrant, left lower quadrant, and left upper quadrant

The second type of question is the fill-in-the-blank question. Traditionally, you may or may not have been given a list of possible responses to fill-in-the-blank questions. When taking a paper-and-pencil exam, you wrote the correct response on the blank line(s). In a computer-based exam, you typed the answer in the appropriate blank in the question. On the NCLEX, *no* possible responses are listed. You will be required to recall the correct response to the fill-in-the-blank questions from memory and to type your answer into the blank space following the question. For an answer to be counted as correct on a fill-in-the-blank question on the computerized NCLEX, the typed responses must be as specific as possible; for example, "aortic," not "aorta." The NCSBN has not determined how multiple varied responses will be handled, but it may not offer a wide variance of responses. At first, until the handling of correct multiple varied responses is determined, most responses will be calculation questions. For example, you may be asked to calculate a client's daily intake and output or a correct medication dose.

Let's practice answering some fill-in-the-blank questions. Remember to be as specific as possible in your responses.

1. What is the cardiac landmark located at the second intercostal space to the right of the sternum called?

Answer: aortic area

2. In what two abdominal quadrants would the nurse assess pain caused from mittelschmerz?

Answer: right lower quadrant and left lower quadrant

The third type of NCLEX alternate question is called an identify-the-area question or "hot spot" question and requires the student to identify an exact area or location on an illustration. This type of question is similar to the traditional illustration-matching questions. The student will be told to place the cursor on the exact spot on the illustration. When completing NCLEX identify-the-area questions, you must place the cursor precisely for the answer to be counted as correct.

Let's practice answering some identify-the-area questions. Remember to be as precise as possible in your responses.

1. The nurse is assessing the S2 sound caused by the closure of the semilunar heart valves. Identify the area where the nurse would place the stethoscope to listen for the closure of the semilunar valves.

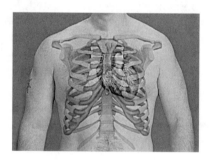

Answer:

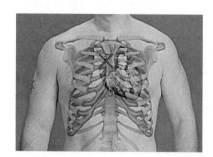

2. A 50-year-old male is admitted with cholecystitis. The results of the endoscopic retrograde cholangiopancreatography confirm the diagnosis. Identify the area of the body affected by cholecystitis.

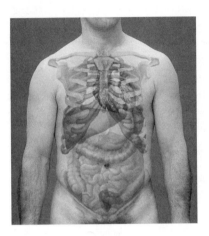

Answer:

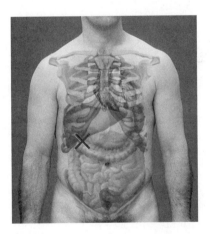

A key to passing the NCLEX-RN is to know the question format and consistently practice NCLEX-style questions throughout your education program. When a student has failed the NCLEX, P. Bostwick, a NCLEX tutor, recommends completing 100 questions a day for 30

days to improve your chance of passing it (personal communication, November 12, 2003). Students have found that routinely practicing NCLEX questions also helps them in taking course exams and being more successful in their courses. It seems to assist the student in critically thinking through questions to obtain the correct response. Several NCLEX review books provide the rationale for the answers to the book's review questions. This knowledge helps you review the background information for the question and assists you in logically analyzing each answer option. If you are not familiar with the rationale for the correct answer, you may need to review the question content further in a textbook.

TEST-TAKING STRATEGIES

Nursing faculty at the State University of West Georgia conducted a research study and developed a course to improve their school's NCLEX-RN scores and assist students in passing the NCLEX-RN. To parallel their program philosophy, the course attempted to integrate the student's body, mind, and spirit. The purpose of the research study was to "increase self-awareness, promote a positive attitude toward passing the NCLEX-RN, and provide specific strategies for test taking and stress reduction" (Mills, Wilson, & Barr, 2001, p. 360).

The university faculty's literature review showed that most programs designed to assist students in passing the NCLEX included test-taking practice and instruction. Students are encouraged to review a set number of questions on a routine basis and then review content in general or content missed on the exam. The literature (Poorman, Webb, Mastorovich, & Molcan, 1999; Saxton, Nugent, & Pelikan, 1999) also supports reviewing the rationale on questions students miss when taking practice tests.

The faculty then designed a course to assist students in passing the NCLEX-RN that included completing a minimum of 1,200 multiple-choice questions and reviewing the rationales for questions they missed. The course also included "cognitive restructuring, relaxation, visualization, and positive self-affirmations" (Mills et al., 2001, p. 361).

According to Mills et al. (2001), "cognitive restructuring focuses on assisting students to understand that cognition, emotion, and behavior are integrated" (p. 367). In other words, what one thinks, how one feels, and how one acts are all intertwined. For example, if a student feels he is not a good test taker he may feel anxious prior to and when taking an exam and consequently receive a lower grade on the exam. If the student's thinking can be changed so that he knows he has some strategies to improve his test-taking skills, the knowledge can decrease his anxiety and result in improved test scores. Or, perhaps as he is taking the exam he comes to a question for which he does not know the content. He may feel his anxiety and negative thoughts returning. If so, he can do self-talk, such as, "I have studied the subject content for this exam. I am not familiar with the content on this question, but that does not mean I will not know the content of other test questions." The student can then relax and concentrate on the rest of the exam. The student needs to learn to recognize prominent, recurring negative thoughts and replace them with factual, positive, and uplifting thoughts.

The State University of West Georgia nursing faculty suggested deep-breathing and shoulder-stretching exercises to assist with relaxation. The students were encouraged to do 30 deep breathing exercises of inhaling for four seconds and then exhaling for eight seconds. They were also encouraged to visualize the testing situation in an effort to desensitize them from the anxiety of the testing situation. Some students included progressive muscle relaxation and music therapy. Progressive muscle relaxation is consciously relaxing a group of muscles and then moving to another set of muscles, until the entire body is relaxed. For example, you can consciously relax tense forehead muscles, then jaw muscles, and so forth. Some students included other relaxation techniques such as lighting candles or taking a warm bath.

The new NCLEX-RN exam will also include analysis, application, delegation, and prioritization questions. An analysis question will include content that needs to be studied, and the information to answer the question will need to be mentally broken down and thought through in order to obtain the correct answer. Do not agonize over the potential answers, but assimilate the information needed to answer the question and mentally review the information learned from hours of study. Rely on what you have learned and know as fact to deduce the correct answer.

To answer an application question correctly, the student must take information he knows and apply it accurately to a clinical situation.

In other words, when answering an application question, the student would ask himself, What do I need to know, and What would I do in a particular clinical situation? For example, if you were shopping and saw an elderly woman fall headfirst on the concrete floor, what information would you have to know, and how would you apply that information to assist the elderly woman? You would need to know the symptoms of brain hemorrhage and possible cervical fracture and assess for these symptoms. You would also need to know appropriate nursing actions. With the background knowledge, you would then choose the best answer option to correctly answer the test question.

Continuing this same scenario with a prioritization question, the student has to decide the best nursing actions to take with the elderly woman. What should the student do first? What should he not do? How should the woman be handled? How should she not be handled? For what symptoms should you assess first, prior to moving her?

The thought process for a delegation question includes these questions: Whom do I need to ask for assistance? Whom do I need to call? To whom can I delegate certain responsibilities? What are the delegatee's abilities?

You will have plenty of opportunity to practice using these thought processes in clinical situations and as you take exams throughout your nursing education experience. By practicing hundreds of NCLEX review questions, you can sharpen your thought processes and be better equipped to successfully take the NCLEX-RN.

Several techniques for success on the NCLEX-RN have been shared here. However, remember that no special techniques can replace knowledge. Practice time management and make reading the textbooks, studying the textbooks' content, and applying your acquired knowledge in the clinical setting a priority in the next few semesters.

The NCLEX-RN will be challenging. Your nursing education has provided you with many opportunities to learn the required content to be successful on the NCLEX-RN. With your new nursing knowledge and knowledge of the new, alternate questions on the NCLEX-RN, you are preparing yourself for success on the NCLEX-RN exam and a successful nursing career.

REFERENCES

Ellis, A., & MacLaren, C. (1998). *Rational emotive behavior therapy: A therapist's guide*. San Luis Obispo, CA: Impact Publishers.

Mills, L., Wilson, C., & Bar, B. (2001). A holistic approach to promoting success on NCLEX-RN. *Journal of Holist Nursing, 19*(4), 360–374.

National Council of State Boards of Nursing (NCSBN). (2003). *Facts about alternate item formats and the NCLEX examinations* [On-line]. Available: http://www.ncsbn.org

Poorman, S., Webb, C., Mastorovich, M., & Molcan, K. (1999). *A good thinking approach to the NCLEX and other nursing exams*. Pittsburgh, PA: STAT Nursing Consultants.

Saxton, D., Nugent, P., & Pelikan, P. (1999). *Mosby's comprehensive review of nursing for NCLEX-RN* (16th ed.). St. Louis, MO: Mosby.

SUGGESTED RESOURCES

Davis, M., Eshelman, E., & McKay, M. (2000). *The relaxation and stress reduction workbook* (5th ed.). Oakland, CA: New Harbinger.

National Council of State Boards of Nursing (NCSBN). (2001). *NCLEX-RN examination test plan for the national council licensure examination for registered nurses* [On-line]. Available: http://www.ncsbn.org

Poorman, S., Mastorovich, M., Webb, C., & Molcan, K. (2002). *Good thinking: Test taking and study skills for nursing students* (2nd ed.). Pittsburgh, PA: STAT Nursing Consultants.

Poorman, S., & Webb, C. (2000). Preparing to take the NCLEX-RN: The experience of graduates who fail. *Nurse Educator, 25*(4), 175–180.

Appendix B
LPN-RN Assessment Skills

▼ ▼ ▼ ▼ ▼ ▼ ▼

As an LPN you are experienced in completing head-to-toe assessments and competent in performing accurate and thorough basic assessments. As you become a registered nursing student, you can refine your assessment skills by learning about or reviewing Gordon's functional health patterns. This assessment method provides a thorough client history and physical assessment. It also assists in adapting client assessments to nursing care plans and the nursing process. We will briefly review Gordon's functional health patterns to assist you in your transition from LPN to RN.

A physical assessment reviews a client's physical state. The nursing health history focuses on the client's response to the illness. A nurse utilizes a health history to provide individualized care, to determine the impact the illness has on the client and the family, to determine health teaching needs, and to begin discharge planning.

Margory Gordon identified functional health patterns to guide data collection and aid in client problem identification. The functional assessment focuses on the psychosocial, physical, and environmental needs and abilities of clients. It determines the abilities of clients to care for themselves. It includes assessment of activities of daily living (ADLs), such as dressing, toileting, and eating. Other aspects of functional assessment include determination of ability to cook, manage finances, and maintain social relationships, along with assessment of self-concept and coping abilities. Gordon's functional health patterns include assessment of:

Health perception/Health management

Nutritional/Metabolic status

Elimination

Activity/Exercise

Sleep/Rest

Cognitive/Perceptual ability

Self-perception/Self-concept

Role relationships

Sexual/Reproductive ability

Coping/Stress tolerance

Values/Beliefs

The functional assessment explores how individuals adjust and acclimate to their present environment. Throughout the performance of a functional assessment, the interviewer's questions focus on the norms and usual environment of the client. These questions assist in establishing what is normal or purposeful to each individual person. This establishes the holistic identification of the client's life and lifestyle.

Topics for questions the nurse can ask within each of the 11 functional health patterns are listed and described in Table B–1. Through use of the topics in the table, the nurse can perform both a health history and a physical examination.

To perform the physical examination or assessment, the nurse may use either a body systems format or a head-to-toe format. When utilizing a body systems approach, the nurse assesses all pertinent information related to a particular body system; for example, the neurological, cardiovascular, or respiratory system. The body systems format can be difficult to remember, whereas in the head-to-toe format the client's body provides a reminder of what should be systematically assessed from head to toe. The physical exam column in Table B–1 does not follow a head-to-toe approach. Rather, the data acquired in the head-to-toe assessment are grouped under specific health patterns to aid in the identification of client problems and nursing diagnoses.

When incorporating a health history within a head-to-toe assessment, the nurse must remember to include answers to questions about the client's habits or usual patterns along with the physical data collected in the assessment. Functional assessment is best done within the framework of the physical assessment because the environment in which each client resides and participates becomes a part of the physical assessment. The functional assessment brings the client's living environment and physical needs together to establish a holistic picture.

Table B–1 Guide sheet for nursing assessment

Health History	Physical Exam
Health Perception/Health Management	

Health History	Physical Exam

• Health perception
  (1) Statement from patient about how patient views overall health
  (2) Statement from patient about why patient is hospitalized
• Lifestyle—Lives:
  Alone or specify with whom
  Type of home
  Nursing home
  No known residence
• Health maintenance:
  Habits: Use of alcohol: none, type and amount per day, week, or month
  Use of tobacco: none, quit date, pipe, cigar, chewing tobacco, cigarettes
    < 1 pack per day, 1–2 packs per day,
    > 2 packs per day
  Other Recreational or OTC Drugs:
  No, yes
  Type
Preventive Health Behaviors:
  Breast or testicular self-examination: yes or no
  Date of last physical examination
  Date of last dental examination
• Problems that could contribute to falls or accidents:
  Age 65 or over
  Confused and disoriented, hallucinating
  History of falls
  Recent history of loss of consciousness, seizure disorder
  Unsteady on feet/physical limitations
  Poor eyesight
  Poor hearing
	• General appearance:
	  Race: Caucasian, black, Hispanic, Asian, other
	  Gender: male, female
	  Age Group: child, teenager, young adult (age), middle aged, elderly
	  Body Build: small, average, large
	  Stature (comparison of height and weight): emaciated, obese, stout, stocky, robust, cachectic, rotund
	  Grooming
	• Signs of distress:
	  Any grossly abnormal signs
	  In acute distress: describe
	  In no acute distress
	• Mental status

Table B–1 (continued)

Health History	Physical Exam
Health Perception/Health Management (continued)	

Drug or alcohol problem

Post-op condition/sedated

Language barrier

Attitude (resistant, belligerent, combative, fearful)

Postural hypotension

• Family history—Risk factors

Nutritional/Metabolic

Health History	Physical Exam
• Previous dietary intake:	• Height and weight:
Diet: Regular, no added salt, ADA, soft, low cholesterol, high fiber, low residue, clear liquids, NPO, list other	• Body temperature:
	• Skin:

• Previous dietary intake:

Diet: Regular, no added salt, ADA, soft, low cholesterol, high fiber, low residue, clear liquids, NPO, list other

Vitamins or Supplements: Name

Food Preferences: List

Appetite: Normal, increased, decreased, presence of nausea or vomiting, decreased taste sensation

• Nutritional impairment:

Inability to swallow (dysphagia): none, to solids or liquids

Inability to chew

Inability to feed self

• Weight fluctuations last 6 months:

None, pounds. Gained/Lost

• Dentures: Upper (partial/full), lower (partial /full)

Usage—describe

• Allergies: List, NKDA

• Skin:

History of Skin/Healing Problems: None, abnormal healing, rash, dryness, pruritus, excess perspiration/diaphoresis

Usual Hygiene Practices: Bath/shower, give frequency

Skin-Care Aids: List

• Height and weight:

• Body temperature:

• Skin:

Color: Light pink to dark pink or light brown to dark brown

Pallor, flushed, cyanotic, ashen, glossy, jaundiced

Color Variations: Erythema, ecchymosis/contusion, petechiae, vitiligo, pigmented

Lesions: Macule, patch

Papule, plaque, nodule, tumor, wheal, verruca, nevus

Vesicle, bulla, pustule, furuncle

Erosion, ulcer, fissure

Crust, scab

Excoration, abrasion, laceration, incisions

Texture: Smooth, soft, rough, thick, scaling

Turgor: Returns immediate/returns > 30 seconds

Temperature and Moisture: Warm, dry, extremely cool, extremely warm, wet, oily

Edema: Absent/0, or 1+, 2+, 3+, 4+

Table B–1 (continued)

Health History	Physical Exam
	Nutritional/Metabolic (continued)

- Hair:
  Color: Describe
  Length: Describe
  Texture: Fine, coarse, pliant, brittle, dull, shiny, lustrous, glossy
  Amount: Thick, thin, normal
  Distribution: Even, alopecia, hirsutism, sparse
- Nails:
  Color: Pink, pale, cyanotic splinter, hemorrhages, poor capillary return
  Shape: Beau's lines, clubbing, spooned
  Texture: Smooth, hard, jagged, soft
  Nail Bed: Smooth, firm, pink, inflamed
- Decubitus risk factor: Calculate and give score
- Mouth:
  Mucous Membranes:
  Color: Pink, pale. cyanotic, reddened
  Consistency: Smooth, moist, dry, bleeding, ulcers, presence of white patches, describe lesions
  Teeth:
  Number: Within normal limits, edentulous
  Position/condition: Stable fixation, smooth surfaces and edges, loose or broken teeth, jagged edges, dental caries, sordes, crooked, protruding, crowded, irregular, broken
  Color: Pearly white and shiny, darkened, brown discoloration
  Gums: Pink, pale, reddened, moist, clearly defined margins, dry, firm, edematous, tenderness, bleeding, ulcers, white patches, receding, shrunken

Table B–1 (continued)

Health History	Physical Exam
	Nutritional/Metabolic (continued)

Health History	Physical Exam
	Tongue: Symmetry/texture: Moist, papillae present, symmetrical appearance, midline fissures, dry, nodules/ulcers present, papillae or fissures absent, asymmetrical, coated, swollen
	• Dietary intake: Regular, no added salt, ADA, soft, low cholesterol, high fiber, low residue, clear liquids, NPO, list other
	Amount Eaten:
	50% or less = poor
	50–75% = fair
	75–100% = good
	• Fluid intake during care:
	Oral: give in cc's
	IV: give in cc's

Elimination	
• Previous Urinary Pattern:	• Urinary:
Frequency of voiding: every____ hours or ____ times/day	Mode: Indwelling catheter, external catheter, incontinence
Problems: Presence of incontinence, dysuria, hematuria, nocturia, urgency, hesitancy	Color: Pale to dark yellow, straw-colored, amber
• Previous Bowel Pattern:	Characteristics: Clear, cloudy, hazy, sediment, aromatic
Number of BMs/day, constipation, diarrhea, incontinence, presence of ostomy	• Bowel/Stool:
Use of laxatives, enemas, suppositories	Bowel Sounds: Audible, hyperactive, hypoactive, inaudible, present, active, not
Last bowel movement	present equally in all quadrants
• Presence of heavy perspiration/ diaphoresis	Abdominal Appearance

Table B–1 (continued)

Health History	Physical Exam
	Elimination (continued)

Contour: Rounded, flat, distended, rotund, scaphoid, enlarged, protruding, hard, rigid, relaxed, taut, pendulous, tympanites

Symmetry: Symmetrical, asymmetrical

Surface motion: no movement, bounding peristalsis, bounding pulsations

- Feces:

Color: Dark brown, medium brown, mustard yellow, green, dark red/bright red, black, tarry, clay-colored

Amount: Small, medium, large

Consistency: Soft, semisolid, formed, hard, loose

Characteristics: Mucoid, foul-smelling, aromatic, pencil-like, bulky, pasty

- Drainage:

Amount: Give in mL's, describe size on dressing

Color: Pink, red, green, brown, white, yellow

Odor: Aromatic, unique, strong

Consistency: Thick, mucoid, watery, thin, frothy, tenacious

Characteristics: Purulent, suppurative, mucopurulent, sanguineous, blood-tinged, serosanguineous, serous

- Emesis:

Hematemesis, bile-colored, amount, contents

- Fluid output during care:

Categorize each type in mL's, then total

Table B–1 (continued)

Health History	Physical Exam
Activity/Exercise	

Health History	Physical Exam
• Previous pattern of activity: Eating/drinking, bathing, dressing/ grooming, toileting, bed mobility, transferring, ambulating, stair climbing, shopping, cooking, home maintenance Rate as independent, use of assistive device, assistance from others, assistance from person and equipment, dependent/ unable • History of tolerance limitations: Pain, stiffness, dyspnea, fatigue, frequent pauses in activity to rest, dizziness • Mobility aids: Crutches, bedside commode, walker, cane, splint/brace, wheelchair, other • Exercise pattern/wellness activities: Type, frequency, length • Limitations in ability: Missing limbs, paralysis, deformities, casts • Vital sign ranges: Either since hospitalization or verbal from patient • Use of diversional activities	• Present pattern of activity: Eating/drinking, bathing, dressing/ grooming, toileting, bed mobility, transferring, ambulating, stair climbing, shopping, cooking, home maintenance. Rate as independent, use of assistive device, assistance from others, assistance from person and equipment, dependent/ unable • Musculoskeletal: Posture: Relaxed, shoulders back, tense, rigid, slumped, asymmetrical posture, kyphosis, lordosis Muscle Tone: Slight resistance, spasticity, rigidity, flaccidity Muscle Strength: Rate all major muscle groups according to the following scale— 0 = No muscular contraction 1 = Barely flicker of contraction 2 = Active movement with gravity removed 3 = Active movement against gravity 4 = Active movement against gravity and some resistance 5 = Active movement against full resistance with no fatigue Gait: Spastic hemiparesis, scissors, steppage, sensory ataxia, cerebellar ataxia, Parkinsonism Balance: Steady, unsteady Range of Motion: Unlimited, full, limited with crepitation or pain, immobile, decreased, restricted Weight Bearing: Give in percentages— ability to stand on left/right heels/toes, weakness, inability to use either extremity

Table B–1 (continued)

Health History	Physical Exam
	Activity/Exercise (continued)

Health History	Physical Exam
	• Cardiorespiratory:
	Lungs:
	Breath sounds: Clear, crackles, rhonchi, wheezes
	Rate: Apneic, eupneic, tachypneic, bradypneic
	Rhythm: Regular, irregular
	Depth: Deep, shallow
	Cough: Continuous, persistent, frequent, productive, nonproductive, spasmodic, paroxysmal, tight, loose, deep, dry, hacking, harsh, painful, rasping, exhaustive
	Use of O_2: Flow rate and method of delivery—mask, nasal cannula
	Heart:
	Rate: Give in numerical value, tachycardic, bradycardic
	Rhythm: Regular, irregular, regularly irregular, irregularly irregular
	Peripheral Vascular:
	BP
	Peripheral pulses: Strong, equal, bounding, thready, imperceptible, weak asymmetrical, absent, 1+, 2+, 3+, 4+
	Sensation: Nontender, can identify light and deep touch, paresthesia, tenderness, pain, tingling, burning, stinging, prickling, numb
	Motor: Hand grasps and foot movement: equal, strong, weakness, paralysis
	• Present tolerance for activity:
	Pain, stiffness, dyspnea, fatigue, frequent pauses in activity to rest, dizziness

Table B–1 (continued)

Health History	Physical Exam
Sleep/Rest	

Health History	Physical Exam

• Sleep patterns: Bedtime, hours slept
  Routine: AM nap, PM nap, work night shifts, variable work*+-shift
• Sleep aids used:
  Medication, food, rituals
• Position of comfort
• Problems:
  None, early waking, insomnia, nightmares
	• Observe appearance: Pale, puffy eyes, dark circles
	• Observe behavior:
	  Yawning, dozing, irritable, short attention span

Cognitive/Perceptual	

Health History	Physical Exam

• Knowledge level
• Educational level achieved
• Primary language spoken
• Developmental level
• Past history of cognitive/perceptual illness
• Past history of sensory perception:
  Heat, cold, taste, smell, touch, vertigo, hearing, sight
• Pain assessment:
  Location, intensity, duration, quality, predisposing factors, grade on 1–10 scale
	• Memory:
	  Long term: Intact, impaired; give example
	  Short term: Intact, impaired; give example
	• Speech:
	  Paralanguage: Qualities of speech—pitch, intonation, rate of speaking, voice volume, words that are stressed or accented
	  Articulation: Articulate, not articulate: describe
	    Sequencing: Logical, illogical: describe
	    Appropriateness of Content: Appropriate, inappropriate
	    Ability to Express Self Verbally: Words or types of expression used
	    Ability to Follow Verbal/Written Instructions: Yes; if no, explain
	• Neurological:
	  Orientation: Person, place, time
	  Pupil Reaction: Sluggish, brisk, PERRLA

Table B-1 (continued)

Health History	Physical Exam
Cognitive/Perceptual (continued)	

Health History	Physical Exam
	Grasp Strength:
	Level of Consciousness: Comatose, unresponsive to verbal or painful stimuli, semiconscious, stuporous, drowsy, lethargic, alert, responsive
	• Perceptual—Cognitive:
	Hallucination: Absent, present
	Delusions: Absent, present
	Attention Span: Intact, not intact: describe
	• Sensory:
	Visual Impairment: Absent, present; describe
	Visual Aids: Absent, present: glasses, contacts, prosthesis
	Auditory Impairment: Absent, present: describe—impaired, deaf, tinnitus
	Auditory Aid: Absent, present
	Other Sensory Impairments: Absent, present: describe
Self-perception/Self-concept	

• Developmental stage of life:
  Give supporting data
• Ability to accomplish age level tasks:
  Describe
• Present health goals:
  Ask the patient: "How would you describe yourself?"
  "What do you consider to be your strengths?"
  Are the goals and responses age related?
• Body image
	• Posture
	• Eye contact:
	  Present, absent: describe
	• Facial expression (affect):
	  Animated, sad, fixed: describe
	• Grooming:
	  Hair groomed: yes, no
	  Hygiene: good, poor: describe
	  Makeup: present, absent
	  Shaven: yes, no
	  Dress: neat, not neat: describe
	• Attitude: Describe
	• Appropriateness of behavior:
	  Appropriate, inappropriate: describe
	• Mood: Describe

Table B–1 (continued)

Health History	Physical Exam
Self-Perception/Self-Concept (continued)	

	• Self-derogatory comments: Present, absent: describe
	• Self-affirmative comments: Present, absent: describe
	• Powerlessness: Present, absent: describe
	• Hopelessness: Present, absent: describe
	• Low self-esteem: Present, absent: describe

Role Relationship

Health History	Physical Exam
• Patterns of relating to others • Identification of own role • Response to authority, peers, subordinates • Age, marital status, occupation • Perceptions of responsibilities in life: Situation at home, work, and in the community	• Observe patient's interaction with others: Verbal, nonverbal communication: describe Does patient have visitors?

Sexuality/Reproductive

Health History	Physical Exam
• Number of living children, abortions, miscarriages, stillbirths • Sexual: self-feelings toward sex, role self-concept • Effect of illness or impairment on sexuality • Present sexual activity • Use of birth control • Age of onset of menses, menopause • Last Pap, mammogram	• Breasts: Round, pendulous, sagging, equal, pink with/without presence of striae Areola: Pink to dark brown, round oval, everted, presence of discharge • Genitalia: Presence and distribution of pubic hair, sexually mature, visible lesions, odor, drainage

Table B–1 (continued)

Health History	Physical Exam
Coping/Stress Tolerance	

• Coping patterns:
  Use of counseling, usual methods of problem solving
• Support system
• Recent loss or change in life situation
• Presence of stress-related disorders
	• Behavior patterns:
	  Abusive to self or others
	  Nervous, relaxed, controlled, agitate, mood swings: describe
	• Appearance
	• Affect
	• Ability to reason and make sound decisions:
	  Able, unable: describe

Value/Belief	

• Health/illness beliefs
• Spiritual, cultural, ethnic heritage, and pattern of participation in
• Concern with meaning of life/death:
  Present, absent: describe
• Concern with meaning of suffering:
  Present, absent: describe
• Anger toward God/religion:
  Present, absent: describe
	• Symbols of faith:
	  Present, absent: describe
	• Current religious/cultural ties:
	  Present, absent: describe (praying, meditation, reading religious materials, clutching religious artifacts, wearing religious jewelry)
	• Visits from clergy

(Courtesy: University of Saint Francis, Ft. Wayne, IN)

Barkauskas, V., Stoltenberg-Allen, K., Baumann, L .& Darling-Fisher, C. (1994). *Health and physical assessment,* St. Louis, Mosby.

Bates, B. (1995). *A guide to physical examination and history taking.* (Sixth ed). Philadelphia: J. B. Lippincott.

Carpenito, L. (1993). *Nursing diagnosis: Application to clinical practice.* (Fifth ed). Philadelphia: J. B. Lippincott.

Cox, H., Hinz, M., Lubno, M., Newfield, S., Ridenour, N., Slater, M., & Sridaromont, K. (1993). *Clinical applications of nursing diagnosis: Adult, child, women's, mental health, gerontic, and home health considerations.* (Second ed). Philadelphia: F. A. Davis.

Taylor, C., Lillis, C., & LeMone, P. (1993). *Fundamentals of nursing: The art and science of nursing care.* (Second ed). Philadelphia: J. B. Lippincott.

From *Medical surgical nursing: An integrated approach,* by L. White, and G. Duncan, Clifton Park, NY: Thomson Delmar Learning.

REFERENCE

Gordon, M. (1995). *Manual of nursing diagnoses 1995–1996* (7th ed.). St. Louis: Mosby–Year Book.

Appendix C
IV Therapy Skills

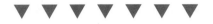

Each of you has a different skill background. The faculty in your LPN-RN program desires to take those skills and mold you into a refined registered nurse. We have presented some basic IV skills that some of you may be very comfortable performing and others may have very little experience. This appendix offers an overview of IV skills to assist you as needed.

ASSESSING THE IV SITE

- Check the health care provider's order for the type of therapy planned to determine the optimal needle size and type to use.
- Know the agency's policy regarding who may start an IV. Many agencies require that nurses have special training before they can perform this procedure.
- Assess the client's veins to optimize planning of the IV site.
- Check the client's fluid, electrolyte, and nutritional status to provide baseline data for comparison with the client's response to IV therapy.
- Assess the client's understanding of the purpose of the procedure so that client teaching can be used to decrease anxiety.

GERIATRIC CONSIDERATIONS

Be careful to use only minimal pressure of the tourniquet because of fragile skin and veins.

Use a 5- to 15-degree angle when inserting the needle because the elderly client's veins are more superficial.

When you tape an IV on an elderly person, try not to use too much tape. Use the least abrasive tape available to reduce irritation to the skin. Be careful when removing the tape as you may pull off skin.

$\mathcal{P}$EDIATRIC CONSIDERATIONS

Using play therapy with a child can assist her in understanding the purpose of IV therapy. Play with the child as she tapes and maintains an IV (without needles) on a doll or teddy bear. As you do, explain what is happening in simple terms appropriate for the child's age. Remind her that this is one of the things nurses do to help sick people get better.

Intravenous pump alarms can cause anxiety and fear in younger and older children. Changing the IV solution is a good opportunity to teach children about the alarms. Remind children that the alarm going off is not an emergency and does not mean that they are in danger or are becoming sicker.

$\mathcal{B}$UTTERFLY NEEDLES

- Butterfly needles are more often used in short-term IV therapy.
- A butterfly needle may be necessary if the client's veins are small or the vein is in a position difficult to access.

$\mathcal{P}$REPARING THE IV BAG AND TUBING

- Check all additives in the solution and other medication so that there will be no incompatibilities with the solution.
- Assess the patency of the IV to ensure that the solution will enter the vein and not the surrounding tissue.
- Assess the skin at the IV site so that the solution will not be administered into an inflamed or edematous site, which could cause injury to the tissue.
- Prepare the new bag by removing its protective cover. Check the expiration date on the bag and assess for cloudiness or leakage.
- Open the new infusion set. Unroll tubing and close roller clamp.
- Spike the bag with the tip of the new tubing and compress the drip chamber to fill half way.
- Open the roller clamp, remove the protective cap from the end of the tubing, and slowly flush solution completely through the tubing. (This process is often called "priming the tubing.")
- Close the roller clamp and replace the cap protector.

- Apply clean gloves.
- Remove the old tubing and replace it with new tubing.
- Discard the old tubing and IV bag.
- Remove gloves and dispose of them with all used materials.
- Apply a label to the tubing with date and time of change. Calculate IV drip rates and begin infusion at the prescribed rate.

SETTING THE IV FLOW RATE

- Check calibration and drops per milliliter (gtt/mL) of each infusion set.

$$\text{Flow Rate} = \frac{\text{Volume} \times \text{Set Calibration}}{\text{Time}}$$

Example:
- The order reads 1000 mL D_5W with 20mEq KCL over 8 hours. Drop factor is 15 gtt/mL

  Divide 1000 mL by 8 hours to obtain 125 mL/hour.

$$\frac{125\,\text{mL}/\,\text{hour} \times 15\,\text{gtts}/\,\text{mL}}{60\,\text{minutes}} = \frac{31.25\,\text{gtts}}{\text{minute}} \text{ or } \frac{31\,\text{gtts}}{\text{minute}}$$

- Determine the hourly rate by dividing total volume by total hours.

Example 1:
- The order reads 1000 mL D_5W with 20mEq KCL over 8 hours:

$$\frac{1000\,\text{ml}}{8\,\text{hrs}} = 125\,\text{mL}/\,\text{hr}$$

Example 2:
- Three thousand milliliters are ordered for 24 hours:

$$\frac{3000\,\text{mL}}{24\,\text{hrs}} = 125\,\text{mL}/\,\text{hr}$$

- Place a strip of tape on the IV bag that identifies the hourly time periods according to the prescribed rate.

- Calculate the number of drops per minute based on the drop factor of the infusion set so you can quickly identify any malfunctioning of the IV pump.

$\mathcal{A}$SSESSING AND MAINTAINING AN IV SITE

- Determine the client's risk for developing complications from IV therapy: being very young or very old, having heart or renal failure, and so forth. Awareness of these risk factors allows for a more focused assessment to better manage any potential complications.
- Observe the IV site for complications such as infection, phlebitis, or infiltration. Signs of these would be redness, swelling, pallor, or warmth at the IV site and surrounding tissue, and bleeding or drainage.
- Teach the client about the purpose of the pump alarm so she will not be concerned or anxious when the alarm sounds.
- Check to make sure you are hanging the prescribed fluid, additives, rate, and volume at the beginning of your shift.
- Check IV tubing for tight connections every four hours.

$\mathcal{D}$ISCONTINUING THE IV AND CHANGING TO A SALINE OR HEPARIN LOCK

- Check the health care provider's order for discontinuation of the IV or insertion of the saline lock.
- If discontinuing an IV and converting to a saline lock, stop IV infusion. Open the sterile package with needleless adapter saline lock. Loosen IV tubing on the existing IV and remove it. Screw saline lock into hub of tubing.

$\mathcal{A}$DMINISTERING MEDICATIONS VIA SECONDARY ADMINISTRATION SETS (PIGGYBACK)

- Check the health care provider's order or the medication administration record (MAR) for the medication, dosage, and time and route of administration to ensure accurate administration.

- Review information regarding the drug, including action, purpose, side effects, normal dose, peak onset, and nursing implications, in order to administer the drug safely.
- Before adding medication to an IV, determine if the additives in the solution of an existing IV line are compatible with the medication.
- Assess the placement of the IV catheter in the vein to ensure that the medication will enter the vein and not the surrounding tissue.
- Check the client's drug allergy history. An allergic reaction could occur rapidly and be fatal.
- Assess the client's understanding of the purpose of the medication so you can tailor teaching to her learning needs.
- Assess the compatibility of the piggyback IV medication with the primary IV solution to avoid an adverse reaction such as the formation of precipitate in the IV tubing.

*I*MPLEMENTATION

- Prepare the medication bag by attaching tubing and filling the tubing with medication.
- Hang the piggyback medication bag above the level of the primary IV bag. One way to do this is to lower the primary bag using an extender; this is often found in the piggyback tubing package.
- Connect the piggyback tubing to the primary tubing at the Y-port.

    For a needleless system, remove cap on port and connect tubing.

    If a needle is used, clean port with antiseptic swab and insert small-gauge needle into center of port. Secure tubing with adhesive tape vertically along the tubing.

SUGGESTED RESOURCES

Altman, G. (2004). *Delmar's fundamental and advanced nursing skills* (2nd ed.). Clifton Park, NY: Thomson Delmar Learning.

Curren, A. (2005). *Math for meds: Dosages and solutions* (9th ed.). Clifton Park, NY: Thomson Delmar Learning.

Appendix D
Medication Preparation and Administration Competency for Registered Nurses

▼ ▼ ▼ ▼ ▼ ▼ ▼

Just the word *math* is enough to frighten some people away from a particular situation. Many people consider themselves math illiterate and live with a math phobia. However, it is inevitable and undisputable that math and nurses must go together. All nurses will administer medications; it does not matter in what area of nursing they choose to practice! There are many situations in the nursing profession that require us to work with numbers and basic calculations, such as measuring daily intakes and outputs, calorie counts, weights, and vital signs; reviewing lab results; and administering medication. Every nurse is expected to be competent in basic math skills for the purpose of administering accurate medication dosages and, most importantly, providing safe care to each client.

PREVENTION OF MEDICATION ERRORS

Situations frequently require the nurse to convert from one system of measurement to another while administering medications. There are many different ways that a medication prescription can be ordered and filled. The nurse may receive an order from the physician written in milligrams, but the pharmacist may supply the medication in grains. In that case, the nurse must be able to convert the ordered dose of medication accurately to verify that the correct dosage is being administered. The rate of medication errors that occur and the consequences of those situations are frightening. Approximately 1.3 million medication errors occur in the United States every year (Karch, 2003). Approximately 44,000 to 98,000 deaths occur every year from medication errors in the United States (Strand, 2003). To put this into perspective, 42,000 people die in traffic accidents each year (Strand). These numbers undeniably indicate the tremendous responsibility nurses have for assuring clients' safety during medication administration. The clients count on us as nurses to be responsible and reliable caregivers.

As nurses, we must take responsibility for our actions. In many cases those errors could have been prevented. Nurses who lack the competency to do dosage calculations in medication preparation and administration present a danger to their clients. The nursing programs you enter will offer you a variety of methods to review and sharpen your skills, but they expect you to come in with a strong understanding of basic math. This appendix serves to reintroduce some of the basic math skills that you may need to understand and use as an RN.

Nursing students make two common errors in dosage calculations (Twiname & Boyd, 2002). The first one is due to errors in basic math skills such as decimals, fractions, and percentages. The second one is misunderstanding the parts of a calculation problem. This might include the extra, or unrelated information, in a scenario to calculate a client's medication dose.

We will review basic medication administration rules and guidelines that should be understood even before any calculations take place. Remember, the "five rights" include: right client, right drug, right dose, right time, and right route. These steps should always be taken in order to prevent medication administration errors. Remember that medications should be checked at least three times while you are preparing to administer them to the client. You also need to know the acceptable abbreviations for weights, values, and measurement conversions in order to administer medications in a competent fashion. These safeguards protect nurses and clients from medication administration errors. They should never be taken lightly.

As you enter your nursing program, it is expected that you can add, subtract, multiply, and divide. A good understanding of ratios and percentages and basic problem-solving skills are also very useful. These basic math skills are the foundation for all dosage calculations in medication preparation and administration in health care today (Pickar, 2004).

$\mathscr{B}$ASIC MATH PRETEST

It is important to know exactly what areas you understand and in what areas you struggle as you decide what to review for dosage-calculation tests. The following 50-question pretest evaluation can indicate where your strengths and areas for improvement lie when dealing with dosage calculations. It will take you approximately an hour and a half to complete this pretest. You will need a piece of scrap paper, a pencil, and a quiet place to work.

Mathematics Pretest Evaluation

Instructions: Carry decimals to the third decimal place and round to the second place. Always express fractions in their lowest possible form.

1. $1517 + 0.63 = $ _____

2. Express the value of $0.7 + 0.035 + 20.006$ rounded to two decimal places. _____

3. $9.5 + 17.06 + 32 + 41.11 + 0.99 = $ _____

4. $\$19.69 + \$304.03 = $ _____

5. $93.2 - 47.09 = $ _____

6. $1005 - 250.5 = $ _____

7. Express the value of $17.156 - 0.25$ rounded to two decimal places. _____

8. $509 \times 38.3 = $ _____

9. $\$4.12 \times 42 = $ _____

10. $17.16 \times 23.5 = $ _____

11. $972 \div 27 = $ _____

12. $2.5 \div 0.001 = $ _____

13. Express the value of $\frac{1}{4} \div \frac{3}{8}$ as a fraction reduced to lowest terms. _____

14. Express $\frac{1500}{240}$ as a decimal._____

15. Express 0.8 as a fraction._____

16. Express $\frac{2}{5}$ as a percentage._____

17. Express 0.004 as a percentage._____

18. Express 5% as a decimal._____

19. Express $33\frac{1}{3}\%$ as a ratio in lowest terms._____

20. Express 1:50 as a decimal._____

21. $\frac{1}{2} + \frac{3}{4} =$_____

22. $1\frac{2}{3} + 4\frac{7}{8} =$_____

23. $1\frac{5}{6} - \frac{2}{9} =$_____

24. Express the value of $\frac{1}{100} \times 60$ as a fraction._____

25. Express the value of $4\frac{1}{4} \times 3\frac{1}{2}$ as a mixed number._____

26. Identify the fraction with the greatest value: $\frac{1}{150}, \frac{1}{200}, \frac{1}{100}$.
_____

27. Identify the decimal with the lowest value:
0.009, 0.19, 0.9._____

28. $\frac{6.4}{0.02} =$_____

29. $\frac{.02+0.16}{.4-0.34} =$_____

30. Express the value of $\frac{3}{12+3} \times 0.25$ as a decimal._____

31. 8% of 50 =_____

32. $\frac{1}{2}\%$ of 18 =_____

33. 0.9% of 24 =_____

Find the value of X. Express your answer as a decimal.

34. $\dfrac{1:1000}{1:100} \times 250 = X$ _____

35. $\dfrac{300}{150} \times 2 = X$ _____

36. $\dfrac{2.5}{5} \times 1.5 = X$ _____

37. $\dfrac{1,000,000}{250,000} \times X = 12$ _____

38. $\dfrac{0.51}{1.7} \times X = 150$ _____

39. $X = (82.4 - 52)\dfrac{3}{5}$ _____

40. $\dfrac{\frac{1}{150}}{\frac{1}{300}} \times 1.2 = X$ _____

41. Express $\frac{2}{10}$ as a fraction in the lowest terms._____

42. Express 2% as a ratio in lowest terms._____

43. If 5 equal medication containers contain 25 tablets total, how many tablets are in each container?_____

44. A person is receiving 0.5 milligrams of a medication four times a day. What is the total amount of medication in milligrams given each day?_____

45. If 1 kilogram equals 2.2 pounds, how many kilograms does a 66-pound child weigh?_____

46. If 1 kilogram equals 2.2 pounds, how many pounds are in 1.5 kilograms? (Express your answer as a decimal.)_____

47. If 1 centimeter equals $\frac{3}{8}$ inch, how many centimeters are in $2\frac{1}{2}$ inches? (Express your answer as a decimal.)_____

48. If 2.5 centimeters equal 1 inch, how long in centimeters is a 3 inch wound? _____

49. This diagnostic test has a total of 50 problems. If you answer 5 problems incorrectly, what percentage will you have answered correctly?_____

50. For every 5 female student nurses in a nursing class, there is 1 male student nurse. What is the ratio of female to male student nurses?_____

(From Pickar, 2004, pp. 2–4).

After completing the pretest, go to the last page of this appendix to check your answers. If you get 43 questions or more correct, you are ready to begin with medication preparation and administration questions. If you get fewer than 43 questions correct, you need to begin some basic math review. This does not mean that you cannot do dosage calculations or that you will make a bad nurse; it simply means you need more practice and, maybe, some help with this component of your education. This pretest assesses your math skills and competency level. It will give you some idea of what areas you need to review in order to be competent and provide safe medication preparation and administration as you progress through your nursing program and your nursing career.

$\mathscr{B}$ASIC MATH FOR REVIEW

A review of fractions and decimals will provide you with a good foundation for solving more complicated calculations.

Adding and Subtracting Fractions

A fraction consists of two numbers (a numerator and a denominator) that identify a portion of another whole number or, figuratively, a piece of the pie. Always write a fraction in its lowest possible form, or terms.

Example:

$$\frac{8}{12} = \frac{2}{3} \text{ or } \frac{25}{50} = \frac{1}{2}$$

To add or subtract fractions, you first need to change the two denominators to the lowest common denominator.

Example:

$$\frac{2}{8}+\frac{1}{2} \text{ becomes } \frac{2}{8}+\frac{4}{8}$$

In the example, 1/2 was changed to 4/8 by multiplying both the numerator and the denominator by 4. Now both fractions share the denominator 8, and you can add them. Last, always reduce the fraction to its lowest possible form.

Example:

$$\frac{2}{8}+\frac{4}{8}=\frac{6}{8} \text{ can be reduced to } \frac{3}{4}$$

Multiplying Fractions

To multiply fractions you first reduce the fractions (when possible), then multiply the numerators together, and then multiply the denominators together. Reduce your answer (the product) to its lowest form.

Example:

$$\frac{125}{250}\times\frac{2}{3}=$$

First, reduce the fractions when possible: $\frac{125}{250}=\frac{1}{2}$; $\frac{2}{3}$ is already in its lowest form. At this point, multiply across the numerators and then multiply across the denominators.

Example:

$$\frac{1\times2}{2\times3}=\frac{2}{6} \text{ (reduced to its lowest form) } \frac{1}{3}$$

To divide fractions, invert the second fraction, or the divisor, and then change *divide* to *multiply*. Cancel or reduce all terms as much as possible. Then, multiply numerators and denominators across. Reduce the answer to its lowest form.

Example:

$$\frac{2}{6}\div\frac{3}{9}=$$

$$\frac{2}{\cancel{6}_{2}}\times\frac{\cancel{9}^{3}}{3}=\frac{6}{6}=1$$

PRACTICE WITH FRACTIONS:

1. Circle all of the fractions that are equal when reduced to their lowest form:

$$\frac{1}{5} = \frac{20}{200} \qquad \frac{2}{6} = \frac{1}{3} \qquad \frac{2}{4} = \frac{1}{2} \qquad \frac{3}{4} = \frac{6}{8} \qquad \frac{33}{66} = \frac{1}{2} \qquad \frac{125}{250} = \frac{2}{3} \qquad \frac{1}{4} = \frac{250}{1000}$$

2. Change the following fractions to whole or mixed numbers (always reduce to the lowest terms).

$$\frac{36}{12} = \underline{\qquad} \qquad \frac{11}{11} = \underline{\qquad} \qquad \frac{66}{33} = \underline{\qquad} \qquad \frac{125}{25} = \underline{\qquad}$$

$$\frac{15}{2} = \underline{\qquad} \qquad \frac{50}{3} = \underline{\qquad}$$

3. Write the following fractions using the specified denominators.

$\frac{2}{4}$ converted to eighths = _____

$\frac{1}{5}$ converted to fifteenths = _____

$\frac{2}{3}$ converted to twelfths = _____

4. A nursing student gets 40 questions correct on a 50-question exam. Write the student's score in a fraction format. Reduce the fraction to its lowest form to show the portion of the exam the student got correct._____

5. In your nursing class there are 5 men and 45 women. What fraction of the students are women? Reduce the fraction to the lowest terms._____

6. Add or subtract the following fractions. Reduce to the lowest form.

$$\frac{2}{4}+\frac{1}{3}= \underline{\hspace{2cm}}$$

$$\frac{2}{4}-\frac{1}{4}= \underline{\hspace{2cm}}$$

$$\frac{1}{5}+\frac{2}{7}= \underline{\hspace{2cm}}$$

$$\frac{6}{8}-\frac{2}{4}= \underline{\hspace{2cm}}$$

$$\frac{3}{9}+\frac{6}{12}= \underline{\hspace{2cm}}$$

$$\frac{3}{6}-\frac{2}{9}= \underline{\hspace{2cm}}$$

7. Multiply or divide the following fractions. Reduce to the lowest form.

$$\frac{3}{8}\times\frac{2}{6}= \underline{\hspace{2cm}}$$

$$\frac{25}{75}\div\frac{2}{5}= \underline{\hspace{2cm}}$$

$$\frac{7}{21}\times\frac{1}{7}= \underline{\hspace{2cm}}$$

$$\frac{11}{33}\div\frac{2}{3}= \underline{\hspace{2cm}}$$

$$\frac{25}{75}\times 6= \underline{\hspace{2cm}}$$

$$\frac{1}{30}\div\frac{2}{3}= \underline{\hspace{2cm}}$$

Decimals

Some key decimal notes are:

Adding zeros after the last digit of a decimal fraction *does not* change its value.

Example:
$$0.50 \text{ is the same as } 0.5$$

Always add a zero to the left of the decimal point to avoid errors and possibly missing the decimal point.

Adding a zero between the decimal point and the first digit of a decimal fraction *does* change its value.

Example:
$$0.05 \text{ is different from } 0.5$$

To convert a fraction to a decimal, divide the numerator by the denominator.

Example:

$$\frac{76}{100} = 76 \div 100 = 0.76$$

To change a decimal to a fraction, write the decimal number as a whole number in the position of the numerator (on top), then write the denominator as the number 1 with as many zeros after it as there were places behind the decimal point. Reduce to the lowest form.

Example:

$$0.125 = \frac{125}{1000} = \frac{1}{8}$$

To add or subtract decimal fractions, simply line up the decimal points and add zeros to make them even.

Example:

$$
\begin{array}{r}
7.250 \\
+32.500 \\
\hline
39.750
\end{array}
$$

When multiplying numbers with decimals, first multiply the numbers and then add the decimal from right to left, one space for each decimal in the original numbers.

Example:

$7.50 \times 12 = 90.00$ or $8.25 \times 2.75 = 22.6875$

(From Pickar, 2004, pp. 26–29.)

PRACTICE WITH DECIMALS

Convert the following numbers to their opposite form in the space provided.

Fraction: $\frac{2}{3}$ _____ $\frac{25}{250}$ _____ $5\frac{1}{3}$ _____

Decimal: 0.95 _____   0.33 _____   1.25 _____

Table D–1 Important conversions

Household measurements	Apothecary system	Metric system
1 tsp	1 dram (60 minims)	4–5 mL
2 tbsp	1 oz (8 drams)	30 mL
1 glass/measuring cup	8 oz	240 mL
1 quart	32 ounces	1,000 mL (1 liter)
15–16 drops	15–16 minims	1 mL
	1 gr	60-65 mg
	15 gr	1 g (1,000 mg)
	1/60 gr	1 mg
1 oz	8 drams	30 grams
1 gtt	1 m	0.06–0.07 mL
2.2 lb		1 kg (1,000 grams)
1 in		2.5 cm

𝒟OSAGE CALCULATION

Once you have completed the necessary review, you are ready to move on to practicing dosage calculation.

Medication Weight, Values, and Measurements

In order to understand and be able to administer the correct dosages of medication, you need to know the different weights, values, and measurements used for medications (see Table D–1). You need to know each system and how to convert between one and another.

Dosage Calculations

If you have established a method or formula for dosage calculations that you understand and that you know consistently produces the correct answers, then by all means, continue to use that method. If not, and if you find that you are one of the many who continue to struggle with and fear dosage calculations, then take this opportunity to grow and develop your math skills for safe medication preparation and administration.

Many people are familiar with the *ratio and proportion* formulas. The formula typically used for this method is:

$$\frac{D \text{ (desired)}}{H \text{ (have)}} \times Q \text{ (quantity)} = X$$

Another method used for calculations is called *dimensional analysis,* or the *factor method.* This is a method that can be used safely with all dosage calculations. In order to use this formula, you need to do the following steps:

1. SETUP: Dimensional analysis problems are set up like fractions. You first must decide what it is that you need to know. You then need to set up the fractions so that the unwanted units of measurement can be canceled out. You continue to write these fractions until all the units present in your question and the ones that you need to find are in your fractions.

2. Next, cross out the units in each fraction that cancel each other out, leaving nothing but the wanted quantity.

3. Finally, do the basic math. Solve the problem by using basic math—no algebra required! Multiply the numbers across the top and then across bottom. Divide the top number by the bottom number. It is as simple as that!

4. When you are done, make sure your answer makes sense. Think about whether the dose should be larger or smaller than what is available. Your answer should always seem realistic. If it does not, recalculate the problem.

Example: The client is to receive 40 mg of Lasix every morning. The dose on hand is 20 mg tablets. How many tablets will the nurse administer?

$$\frac{\text{Tabs}}{\text{Dose}} = \frac{1 \text{ tab}}{20 \text{ mg}} \times \frac{40 \text{ mg}}{\text{dose}} = \frac{40 \text{ tabs}}{20 \text{ mg dose}} = \frac{2 \text{ tabs}}{\text{dose}}$$

Example: The client is to receive 500 mg of X drug q 4h. The label reads "1gram/5mL." How many mL will the nurse administer per dose?

$$\frac{\text{mL}}{\text{Dose}} = \frac{5 \text{ mL}}{1 \text{ mg}} \times \frac{1 \text{ gm}}{1,000 \text{ mg}} \times \frac{500 \text{ mg}}{\text{dose}} = \frac{5}{2} = \frac{2.5 \text{ mL}}{\text{dose}}$$

Example: The physician orders 125 mL/hour of 5% dextrose in water with 40 mEq of kcl. The drop factor for the IV administration tubing is

15 gtt/mL. The nurse will correctly set the drip rate to run at how many drops per minute?

$$\frac{gtt}{min} = \frac{15\,gtt}{1\,mL} \times \frac{125\,mL}{1\,hr} \times \frac{1\,hr}{60\,min} = 31.25 \text{ which rounds to } 31\,\frac{gtt}{min}$$

PRACTICE WITH DOSAGE CALCULATIONS

1. The physician has ordered 0.25 mg digoxin. You have available 0.125 mg tablets. How many tablets will you give? _____

2. Coumadin 10 mg is prescribed. You have available 2.5 mg tablets. How many tablets will you give? _____

3. Dilantin 300 mg is prescribed. You have available Dilantin suspension 125 mg/5 cc. How many mL will you give? _____

4. Motrin 0.8 g is prescribed. Motrin 400 mg tablets are available. How many tablets will you give? _____

5. Tylenol gr X is prescribed. You have available Tylenol Elixer labeled 160 mg/teaspoon. How many mL will you give? _____

6. Nitroglycerin grains 1/150 is prescribed. Nitroglycerin 0.4 mg tablets are available. How many tablets will you give? _____

7. Diabeta 5 mg is ordered. You have available 1.25 mg tablets. How many tablets will you give? _____

8. Demerol 35 mg IM was ordered for pain. Demerol is available in 50 mg/mL. How many mL will you administer? _____

9. Versed 3 mg IM was ordered pre-op. You have available Versed 2 mg/mL. How many mL will you administer IM? _____

10. The nurse practitioner ordered 125 mg of Solu-Medrol IM for severe inflammation. Powder in a 0.5 gram vial is available. You would reconstitute it according to the vial directions so that each 8 mL will contain 0.5 grams of Solu-Medrol. How many mL will you give in order to give 125 mg? _____

11. The physician prescribed 25 mg of Librium IM. You will need to add 2 cc diluent to make it 100 mg/2 mL. How many mL will you give? _____

12. The physician prescribed Primaxin 600 mg IM every 12 hours. The drug available is 750 mg/mL. How many mL will you give?

_____

$\mathcal{S}$UMMARY

The general rule of thumb is to practice, practice, and practice. When students and nurses stop using these math skills they begin to lose their confidence, competency skills, and comprehension of the dosage calculation process. Brown (2002) believes that an emphasis on math should be put into real-life situations whenever the opportunity arises to better develop medication administration competency skills. In your nursing clinicals, you should take every opportunity afforded you to practice dosage calculation problems, even when the calculations have already been done for you by the pharmacy. Use your time with mentors to discuss your problem areas and do problem solving together. As your understanding of dosage calculations grows, so too will your confidence, your competence, and the safety of your clients. Always remember, safety first! But remember too that mistakes can and do happen. Everyone is human and can err in this process. Placing blame is easy, but accepting the consequences and responsibility for errors and moving forward to find solutions to prevent them from recurring takes accountability and dedication to your clients and to the nursing profession (Swihart, 2004).

$\mathcal{B}$ASIC MATHEMATICS PRETEST EVALUATION ANSWER KEY

1) 1517.63

2) 20.74

3) 100.66

4) $323.72

5) 46.11

6) 754.5

7) 16.91

8) 19,494.7

9) $173.04

10) 403.26

11) 36

12) 2500

13) $\frac{2}{3}$

14) 6.25

15) $\frac{4}{5}$

16) 40%

17) 0.4%

18) 0.05

19) 1:3

35) 4

20) 0.02

36) 0.75

21) $1\frac{1}{4}$

37) 3

22) 6 13/24

38) 500

23) $1\frac{11}{18}$

39) 18.24

24) 3/5

40) 2.4

25) $14\frac{7}{8}$

41) $\frac{1}{5}$

26) $\frac{1}{100}$

42) 1:50

27) 0.009

43) 5 tablets

28) 320

44) 2 milligrams

29) 3

45) 30 kilograms

30) 0.05

46) 3.3 pounds

31) 4

47) $6\frac{2}{3} = 6.67$ centimeters

32) 0.09

48) 7.5 centimeters

33) 0.22

49) 90%

34) 25

50) 5:1

$\mathscr{P}$RACTICE WITH FRACTIONS ANSWER KEY

1. Circled are $\frac{2}{6} = \frac{1}{3}$, $\frac{2}{4} = \frac{1}{2}$, $\frac{3}{4} = \frac{6}{8}$, $\frac{33}{66} = \frac{1}{2}$, and $\frac{1}{4} = \frac{250}{1000}$

2. 3, 1, 2, 5, $7\frac{1}{2}$, and $16\frac{2}{3}$

3. $\frac{4}{8}$, $\frac{3}{15}$, and $\frac{8}{12}$

4. $\dfrac{4}{5}$

5. $\dfrac{9}{10}$

6. Addition column is $\dfrac{5}{6}$, $\dfrac{17}{35}$, and $\dfrac{5}{6}$; subtraction column is $\dfrac{1}{4}$, $\dfrac{1}{4}$ and $\dfrac{5}{18}$

7. Multiplication column is $\dfrac{1}{8}$, $\dfrac{1}{21}$, and 3; division column is $\dfrac{5}{6}$, $\dfrac{1}{2}$ and $\dfrac{1}{20}$

$\mathscr{P}$RACTICE WITH DECIMALS ANSWER KEY

Fraction row: $\dfrac{95}{100}$, $\dfrac{33}{100}$, and $\dfrac{125}{100}$

Decimal row: 0.66, 0.1, and 5.33

$\mathscr{P}$RACTICE WITH DOSAGE CALCULATIONS ANSWER KEY

1. 2 tablets
2. 4 tablets
3. 12 mL
4. 2 tablets
5. 2 tsp
6. 1 tablet
7. 4 tablets
8. 0.7 mL
9. 1.5 mL
10. 2 mL
11. 0.5 mL
12 .0.8 mL

REFERENCES

Brown, D. (2002). Does 1+1 still equal 2? A study of the mathematic competencies of associate degree nursing students. *Nurse Educator, 27*(3), 132–135.

Karch, A. (2003). *Lippincott's guide to preventing medication errors.* Philadelphia: Lippincott Williams & Wilkins.

Pickar, G. (2004). *Dosage calculations* (7th ed.). Clifton Park, NY: Thomson Delmar Learning.

Strand, R. D. (2003). *Death by prescription.* Nashville, TN: Thomas Nelson Publishers.

Swihart, D. (2004). First do no harm: Preventing medical errors. *Advance Online.* Retrieved December 21, 2003, from http://www.advancefornurses. com/common/editorial/editorial

Twiname, B., & Boyd, S. (2002). *Student nurse handbook: Difficult concepts made easy* (2nd ed.). Upper Saddle River, NJ: Prentice Hall.

Woods, A. (2003). Patient safety: Not a question of competencies. *Nursing Management, 34*(9), 6.

SUGGESTED RESOURCES

Curren, A. (2002). Dimensional analysis for meds (2nd ed.). Clifton Park, NY: Thomson Delmar Learning.

Curren, A. (2005). Math for meds: Dosages and solutions (9th ed.). Clifton Park, NY: Thomson Delmar Learning.

Indiana State University. *ISU Nursing Mini Math Tutorial* [On-line]. Available: www-isu.indstate.edu/nurs/mary/tutorial.htm

Math Magic for Meds. [On-line]. Available: www.edgt.com

Appendix E
American Nurses Association
Code of Ethics

▼ ▼ ▼ ▼ ▼ ▼ ▼

APPROVED AS OF JUNE 30, 2001

The ANA House of Delegates approved these nine provisions of the new *Code of Ethics for Nurses* at its June 30, 2001, meeting in Washington, DC. In July 2001, the Congress of Nursing Practice and Economics voted to accept the new language of the interpretive statements resulting in a fully approved revised *Code of Ethics for Nurses with Interpretive Statements.*

1. The nurse, in all professional relationships, practices with compassion and respect for the inherent dignity, worth, and uniqueness of every individual, unrestricted by considerations of social or economic status, personal attributes, or the nature of health problems.

2. The nurse's primary commitment is to the patient, whether an individual, family, group, or community.

3. The nurse promotes, advocates for, and strives to protect the health, safety, and rights of the patient.

4. The nurse is responsible and accountable for individual nursing practice and determines the appropriate delegation of tasks consistent with the nurse's obligation to provide optimum patient care.

5. The nurse owes the same duties to self as to others, including the responsibility to preserve integrity and safety, to maintain competence, and to continue personal and professional growth.

6. The nurse participates in establishing, maintaining, and improving healthcare environments and conditions of employment conducive to the provision of quality health care and consistent

with the values of the profession through individual and collective action.

7. The nurse participates in the advancement of the profession through contributions to practice, education, administration, and knowledge development.

8. The nurse collaborates with other health professionals and the public in promoting community, nation, and international efforts to meet health needs.

9. The profession of nursing, as represented by associations and their members, is responsible for articulating nursing values, for maintaining the integrity of the profession and its practice, and for shaping social policy.

Reprinted with permission from American Nurses Association, *Code of Ethics for Nurses with Interpretive Statements,* ©2001 American Nurses Publishing, American Nurses Association, Washington, DC.

$\mathscr{A}$ppendix F
The International Council
of Nurses Code of Ethics

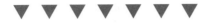

An international code of ethics for nurses was first adopted by the International Council of Nurses (ICN) in 1953. It has been revised and reaffirmed at various times since, most recently with this review and revision completed in 2000. The ICN Code of Ethics is also available in French [pdf file], Spanish [pdf file], and German.

$\mathscr{P}$REAMBLE

Nurses have four fundamental responsibilities: to promote health, to prevent illness, to restore health and to alleviate suffering. The need for nursing is universal.

Inherent in nursing is respect for human rights, including the right to life, to dignity and to be treated with respect. Nursing care is unrestricted by considerations of age, colour, creed, culture, disability or illness, gender, nationality, politics, race or social status.

Nurses render health services with those of related groups.

$\mathscr{T}$HE CODE

The *ICN Code of Ethics* has four principal elements that outline the standards of ethical conduct.

Elements of the Code

1. Nurses and people

   The nurse's primary professional responsibility is to people requiring nursing care.

In providing care, the nurse promotes an environment in which the human rights, values, customs and spiritual beliefs of the individual, family and community are respected.

The nurse ensures that the individual receives sufficient information on which to base consent for care and related treatment.

The nurse holds in confidence personal information and uses judgement in sharing this information.

The nurse shares with society the responsibility for initiating and supporting action to meet the health and social needs of the public, in particular those of vulnerable populations.

The nurse also shares responsibility to sustain and protect the natural environment from depletion, pollution, degradation and destruction.

2. Nurse and practice

The nurse carries personal responsibility and accountability for nursing practice, and for maintaining competence by continual learning.

The nurse maintains a standard of personal health such that the ability to provide care is not compromised.

The nurse uses judgement regarding individual competence when accepting and delegating responsibility.

The nurse at all times maintains standards of personal conduct which reflect well on the profession and enhance public confidence.

The nurse, in providing care, ensures that use of technology and scientific advances are compatible with the safety, dignity and rights of people.

3. Nurses and the profession

The nurse assumes the major role in determining and implementing acceptable standards of clinical nursing practice, management, research and education.

The nurse is active in developing a core of research-based professional knowledge.

The nurse, acting through the professional organisation, participates in creating and maintaining equitable social and economic working conditions in nursing.

4. Nurse and co-workers

The nurse sustains a co-operative relationship with co-workers in nursing and other fields.

The nurse takes appropriate action to safeguard individuals when their care is endangered by a co-worker or any other person.

SUGGESTIONS FOR USE OF THE *ICN CODE OF ETHICS*

The *ICN Code of Ethics* is a guide for action based on social values and needs. It will have meaning only as a living document if applied to the realities of nursing and health care in a changing society.

To achieve its purpose the *Code* must be understood, internalised and used by nurses in all aspects of their work. It must be available to students and nurses throughout their study and work lives.

APPLYING THE ELEMENTS OF THE *ICN CODE OF ETHICS*

The four elements of the *ICN Code of Ethics:* nurses and people, nurses and practice, nurses and co-workers, and nurses and the profession, give a framework for the standards of conduct. The following chart will assist nurses to translate the standards into action. Nurses and nursing students can therefore:

- Study the standards under each element of the *Code.*
- Reflect on what each standard means to you. Think about how you can apply ethics in your nursing domain: practice, education, research or management.
- Discuss the *Code* with co-workers and others.
- Use a specific example from experience to identify ethical dilemmas and standards of conduct as outlined in the *Code.* Identify how you would resolve the dilemma.
- Work in groups to clarify ethical decision making and reach a consensus on standards of ethical conduct.

- Collaborate with your national nurses' association, co-workers, and others in the continuous application of ethical standards in nursing practice, education, management and research.

Element of the Code #1: Nurses and People

Practitioners and Managers	Educators and Researchers	National Nurses' Associations
Provide care that respects human rights and is sensitive to the values, customs and beliefs of people.	In curriculum include references to human rights, equity, justice, solidarity as the basis for access to care.	Develop position statements and guidelines that support human rights and ethical standards.
Provide continuing education in ethical issues.	Provide teaching and learning opportunities for ethical issues and decision making.	Lobby for involvement of nurses in ethics review committees.
Provide sufficient information to permit informed consent and the right to choose or refuse treatment.	Provide teaching/learning opportunities related to informed consent.	Provide guidelines, position statements and continuing education related to informed consent.
Use recording and information management systems that ensure confidentiality.	Introduce into curriculum concepts of privacy and confidentiality.	Incorporate issues of confidentiality and privacy into a national code of ethics for nurses.
Develop and monitor environmental safety in the workplace.	Sensitise students to the importance of social action in current concerns.	Advocate for safe and healthy environment.

Element of the Code #2: Nurses and Practice

Practitioners and Managers	Educators and Researchers	National Nurses' Associations
Establish standards of care and a work setting that promotes quality care.	Provide teaching/learning opportunities that foster lifelong learning and competence for practice.	Provide access to continuing education, through journals, conferences, distance education, etc.
Establish systems for professional appraisal, continuing education and systematic renewal of licensure to practice.	Conduct and disseminate research that shows links between continual learning and competence to practice.	Lobby to ensure continuing education opportunities and quality care standards.
Monitor and promote the personal health of nursing staff in relation to their competence for practice.	Promote the importance of personal health and illustrate its relation to other values.	Promote healthy lifestyles for nursing professionals. Lobby for healthy workplaces and services for nurses.

Element of the Code #3: Nurses and the Profession

Practitioners and Managers	Educators and Researchers	National Nurses' Associations
Set standards for nursing practice, research, education and management.	Provide teaching/learning opportunities in setting standards for nursing practice, research, education and management.	Collaborate with others to set standards for nursing education, practice, research and management.
Foster workplace support of the conduct, dissemination and utilisation of research related to nursing and health.	Conduct, disseminate and utilise research to advance the nursing profession.	Develop position statements, guidelines and standards related to nursing research.
Promote participation in national nurses' associations so as to create favourable socio-economic conditions for nurses.	Sensitise learners to the importance of professional nursing associations.	Lobby for fair social and economic working conditions in nursing. Develop position statements and guidelines in workplace issues.

Element of the Code #4: Nurses and Co-workers

Practitioners and Managers	Educators and Researchers	National Nurses' Associations
Create awareness of specific and overlapping functions and the potential for interdisciplinary tensions.	Develop understanding of the roles of other workers.	Stimulate co-operation with other related disciplines.
Develop workplace systems that support common professional ethical values and behaviour.	Communicate nursing ethics to other professions.	Develop awareness of ethical issues of other professions.
Develop mechanisms to safeguard the individual, family or community when their care is endangered by health care personnel.	Instill in learners the need to safeguard the individual, family or community when care is endangered by health care personnel.	Provide guidelines, position statements and discussion for a related to safeguarding people when their care is endangered by health care personnel.

𝒟ISSEMINATION OF THE *ICN CODE OF ETHICS*

To be effective the *ICN Code of Ethics* must be familiar to nurses. We encourage you to help with its dissemination to schools of nursing, practising nurses, the nursing press and other mass media. The *Code* should also be disseminated to other health professions, the general public, consumer and policy making groups, human rights organisations and employers of nurses.

𝒢LOSSARY OF TERMS USED IN THE *ICN CODE OF ETHICS*

Co-operative relationship	A professional relationship based on collegial and reciprocal actions, and behaviour that aim to achieve certain goals.
Co-worker	Other nurses and other health and non-health related workers and professionals.
Nurse shares with society	A nurse, as a health professional and a citizen, initiates and supports appropriate action to meet the health and social needs of the public.
Personal health	Mental, physical, social and spiritual well-being of the nurse.
Personal information	Information obtained during professional contact that is private to an individual or family, and which, when disclosed, may violate the right to privacy, cause inconvenience, embarrassment, or harm to the individual or family.
Related groups	Other nurses, health care workers or other professionals providing service to an individual, family or community and working toward desired goals.

*A*ppendix G
National Student Nurses' Association, Inc.
Code of Professional Conduct

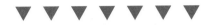

As a member of the National Student Nurses' Association, I pledge myself to:

- Maintain the highest standard of personal and professional conduct.
- Actively promote and encourage the highest level of ethics within nursing education, the profession of nursing, and the student nurses' association.
- Uphold all Bylaws and regulations relating to the student nurses' association at the chapter, state and national levels, reserving the right to criticize rules and laws constructively, but respecting the rules and laws as long as they prevail.
- Strive for excellence in all aspects of decision making and management at all levels of the student nurses' association.
- Use only legal and ethical principles in all association decisions and activities.
- Ensure the proper use of all association funds.
- Serve all members of the student nurses' association impartially, provide no special privilege to any individual member, and accept no personal compensation from another member or non-member.
- Maintain the confidentiality of privileged information entrusted or known to me by virtue of an elected or appointed position in the association.
- Refuse to engage in, or condone, discrimination on the basis of race, gender, age, citizenship, religion, national origin, sexual orientation, or disability.
- Refrain from any form of cheating or dishonesty, and take action to report dishonorable practices to proper authorities using established channels.

- Always communicate internal and external association statements in a truthful and accurate manner by ensuring that there is integrity in the data and information used by the student nurses' association.

- Cooperate in every reasonable and proper way with association volunteers and staff, and work with them in the advocacy of student rights and responsibilities and the advancement of the profession of nursing.

- Use every opportunity to improve faculty understanding of the role of the student nurses association.

- Use every opportunity to raise awareness of the student nurses' association's mission, purpose, and goals at the school chapter level.

- Promote and encourage entering nursing students to join and become active in NSNA.

- Promote and encourage graduating seniors to continue their involvement by joining professional nurses' associations upon licensure as Registered Nurses.

Reprinted by permission, National Student Nurses' Association, Inc. 45 Main Street, Suite 606, Brooklyn, New York, 11201, www.nsna.org. Adopted by the 1999 National Student Nurses' Association House of Delegates Pittsburgh, PA at the 47th Annual NSNA Convention.

REFERENCES

American Society of Association Executives and the National Society for Fund Raising Executives.

Appendix H
National Student Nurses' Association, Inc.
Code of Academic and Clinical Conduct

▼ ▼ ▼ ▼ ▼ ▼ ▼

PREAMBLE

Students of nursing have a responsibility to society in learning the academic theory and clinical skills needed to provide nursing care. The clinical setting presents unique challenges and responsibilities while caring for human beings in a variety of health care environments.

The Code of Academic and Clinical Conduct is based on an understanding that to practice nursing as a student is an agreement to uphold the trust with which society has placed in us. The statements of the Code provide guidance for the nursing student in the personal development of an ethical foundation and need not be limited strictly to the academic or clinical environment but can assist in the holistic development of the person.

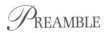 CODE FOR NURSING STUDENTS

As students are involved in the clinical and academic environments we believe that ethical principles are a necessary guide to professional development. Therefore within these environments we:

Advocate for the rights of all clients.

Maintain client confidentiality.

Take appropriate action to ensure the safety of clients, self, and others.

Provide care for the client in a timely, compassionate and professional manner.

Communicate client care in a truthful, timely and accurate manner.

Actively promote the highest level of moral and ethical principles and accept responsibility for our actions.

Promote excellence in nursing by encouraging lifelong learning and professional development.

Treat others with respect and promote an environment that respects human rights, values and choice of cultural and spiritual beliefs.

Collaborate in every reasonable manner with the academic faculty and clinical staff to ensure the highest quality of client care

Use every opportunity to improve faculty and clinical staff understanding of the learning needs of nursing students.

Encourage faculty, clinical staff, and peers to mentor nursing students.

Refrain from performing any technique or procedure for which the student has not been adequately trained.

Refrain from any deliberate action or omission of care in the academic or clinical setting that creates unnecessary risk of injury to the client, self, or others.

Assist the staff nurse or preceptor in ensuring that there is full disclosure and that proper authorizations are obtained from clients regarding any form of treatment or research.

Abstain from the use of alcoholic beverages or any substances in the academic and clinical setting that impair judgment.

Strive to achieve and maintain an optimal level of personal health.

Support access to treatment and rehabilitation for students who are experiencing impairments related to substance abuse and mental or physical health issues.

Uphold school policies and regulations related to academic and clinical performance, reserving the right to challenge and critique rules and regulations as per school grievance policy.

Index

▼ ▼ ▼ ▼ ▼ ▼ ▼

A